RIDE YOUR WAY LEAN

THE ULTIMATE PLAN FOR BURNING FAT AND GETTING FIT ON A BIKE

SELENE YEAGER

AND THE EDITORS OF **Bicycling**.

RODALE

© 2010 by Selene Yeager

Rodale books may be purchased for business or promotional use or for special sales. For information, please write to:

Special Markets Department, Rodale Inc., 733 Third Avenue, New York, NY 10017

Printed in the United States of America

Rodale Inc. makes every effort to use acid-free ♾, recycled paper ♻.

Photographs by Thomas MacDonald/Rodale Images

Book design by Joanna Williams

Library of Congress Cataloging-in-Publication Data

Yeager, Selene.
    Ride your way lean : the ultimate plan for burning fat and getting fit on a bike / by Selene Yeager.
        p.   cm.
    Includes index.
    ISBN-13 978–1–60529–406–3   paperback
    ISBN-10 1–60529–406–3   paperback
    1. Cycling—Health aspects.   2. Cycling—Physiological aspects.   3. Physical fitness.
    4. Weight loss.   I. Title.
    RC1220.C8Y43 2010
    613.7′11—dc22

                                                                                    2010014430

Distributed to the trade by Macmillan

    4   6   8   10   9   7   5   3   paperback

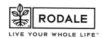

This book is for Dave: not because he needs to lose weight, but because he carries so much of it while I work, train, and race. Without you, it would be too much for me to bear. Thanks.

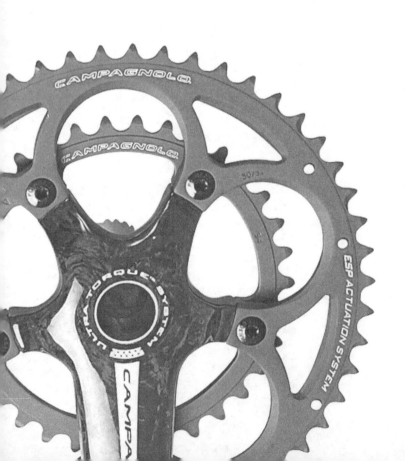

CONTENTS

ACKNOWLEDGMENTS

It takes a village to write a book. I'm fortunate enough to have a great one. First, I'd like to thank my family, who generously give me all the time I need to research, write, and train. It's not always easy, but they always make it happen. Thanks, Dave, Juniper, and my mom and dad. None of this happens without you. On the professional side, thank you to James Herrera, my right-hand man who is always ready with some brilliant programming; Loren Mooney for the early reads and great recommendations; Denise McGann for stepping in and so seamlessly taking the reins; Joanna Williams for her sharp photography and design eye; Mike Cushionbury and Ron Koch for the tech-talk assistance; Tim Church, Leslie Bonci, Cynthia Sass, Andy Pruitt, and the many nutritionists, coaches, and researchers who are always willing to pick up the phone and impart their wisdom; and to all the readers and fellow riders who shared their stories. This book is for all of you.

INTRODUCTION

RIDE IT OFF

FIRST, A CONFESSION. Though I've carried the "Fit Chick" moniker now for 10 years, it's not always been smooth sailing to stay fit over that time. In fact, I'll never forget my own personal "lightbulb" moment, when I realized my weight was creeping out of control. I'd just moved to Emmaus, Pennsylvania, where *Bicycling* is published. I was at the pool, doing some cross-training, dreaming about maybe doing a triathlon one day. Bill Humphreys, a former pro roadie, was there too. He worked on the advertising side at the magazine at the time. We'd been riding together, and he was clearly frustrated with me.

"You'd crush those climbs if you just dropped 10 pounds," he groused with all the tender subtlety of Burgess Meredith playing coach to Rocky Balboa. *Ouch.* I knew I was no whippet. But I'd been riding lots, lifting weights, swimming, and running. I'd just accepted that I was a big girl. At that moment, sitting suddenly terribly self-consciously in my Speedo at the community pool, I brushed him off and basically told him where to go. But deep inside, I wondered if he wasn't right.

Turns out, of course, he was. Like so many cyclists (and regular exercisers), I thought I was doing all the right things. I mean, I was a professional fitness trainer. I *knew* all the right things. But in the end, I was making the same mistakes I've seen (and even preached against) a million times. I had zero structure. I'd just ride around on my bike, swim a few laps, run the same speed time and time again on the cinder path. I overestimated what I burned and buried myself in carbs (more on that later). Once I corrected those errors—and it actually didn't take all that much—10 pounds came off. And stayed off. My climbing performance? Yeah, that took off too.

Does losing 10 pounds qualify me to write a book on weight loss? By itself, no. But over the years I, along with my great friend and colleague James Herrera of Performance Driven consulting in Colorado Springs, Colorado (who penned the plans you'll find in later chapters), have counseled countless clients on how to shed pounds—lots of them—using the advice in this book. I've also pored over reams of research and interviewed dozens of riders and coaches who have won the battle of the bulge with a bike. I can say with complete conviction, whether you have a little or a lot of weight to lose, cycling is the perfect vehicle by which to do it, because it offers a unique benefit for everyone.

✳INSTANT GRATIFICATION, LONG-TERM RESULTS

Take Scott Harris. At 38, he knew he'd put on some weight. It was to be expected, right? He's married, has four kids, and works insane hours in a high-stress job at a software company in American Fork, Utah. A guy's bound to pack on a few pounds by his mid-thirties. But then in a picture with his brand-new fourth child, he got a glimpse of what he really looked like. It stopped him in his tracks. "I usually avoid being in pictures. This time someone caught me and I couldn't believe what I saw. I was shockingly big—285 pounds to be exact. I decided right there and then to change. I started running, because I figured that's what you do. And I lost 15 pounds. But my knee was killing me. I thought, 'I need to get a bike.'" Fresh tax refund in hand, Scott convinced his wife that a road bike was the answer.

He loved it. Not just for the fun and the pain-free freedom, but also because he could really track his progress on a bike. "I'm an analyst. I love numbers. So I got a heart rate monitor and cycling computer and started tracking and charting. I would do a 12- to 15-mile loop around my house in about 40 or 50 minutes and would be completely gassed by the end. So I made it my goal to shave time from that loop; and when I did, I added distance and elevation. I really liked it. Riding is so much faster than running, and you can cover so much territory in a short time. It's energizing and relaxing all at the same time," says Scott, who now regularly rides centuries (100-mile bike rides) and weighs in at a healthy 180 pounds. "My life is so much better because of cycling. It's the best thing I've done for myself."

Then there's Elizabeth Potter, 27, a single mom, bike racer, and former emotional eater from Salt Lake City, Utah, who tipped the scales at 255 pounds when she was in her early twenties. For the longest time she never even tried to lose weight. She simply avoided mirrors and "self-medicated" with food. "I'm a single mom and I just thought, 'There's no way. I can't afford a sitter so I can go exercise.' I couldn't afford an expensive gym membership. It just seemed futile." Then one day she'd had enough. She knew she needed to lose weight if she wanted to be a healthy mom, and she knew she needed to find something she could do with her son, since she didn't have daycare. So she decided to buy a bike.

"I walked into our local sporting goods store and bought the least expensive mountain bike I could find ($475 to be exact). It was extremely heavy, but it had to do. I needed to take my son with me, so I bought a trailer too. That first ride was just humorous. There I was trying my hardest to pull my son in a trailer with headwinds blowing us backwards. I felt like I was climbing Mount Everest on a flat surface." Elizabeth kept pedaling, 7 days a week, even during Utah's cold winter months. She didn't even have the proper clothes, but she didn't care, because it was working. As she lost weight, the mountain felt smaller and her joy grew bigger. "My friend felt sorry for me because he saw how cold and unprepared I was," she recalls. "He loaned me his arm and leg warmers and shoe covers. He also told me about padded cycling pants and jerseys and clipless pedals."

The love of the sport grew with her knowledge of it. "I started watching the Tour de France, and something inside just clicked. I loved how it felt to ride. I wanted to ride fast and far like that." A year after that first challenging outing "up Everest," Elizabeth walked into the same shop and bought a road bike that weighed less than 17 pounds.

"I went from riding 15 miles on a mountain bike to doubling it on the road, challenging myself to ride 40 to 50 through the canyons. The transition was a little difficult, learning about shifting and braking, but I loved it," she recalls. Her family was so impressed, her mom offered to watch her son so that she would have more time to ride. Two years later, holding steady at 150 pounds, Elizabeth started entering (and winning) local road races. "It's changed my life. I used to eat whatever and whenever, lots of soda and fast food. But once I began to cycle, my diet changed dramatically. Food became energy for riding. I started cooking healthy meals and snacking on nuts and vegetables. I'm not completely strict these days, but I haven't gained the weight back. I know I'll never be the person I was before I took up cycling, because I've found my passion, and that lasts a lifetime."

How's that for a couple of big losers? Both of them with triple-digit weight loss, simply by falling in love with a bike. They're far from isolated examples. At *Bicycling* magazine, where I write the Fit Chick column each month, we receive dozens of stories just like this from readers who haven't lost just a few pounds or dropped a dress size, but who have literally shed the weight of a second person—leaving behind 100 pounds or more—by discovering the joy of cycling.

BIG LOSERS ON BIKES

It kills me to watch *The Biggest Loser* and have them never promote cycling as an ideal way to lose weight. Sure, you'll see contestants on a Spin bike at the gym, cranking away and soaking their shirts. But I feel like screaming at the TV (well, sometimes I actually do scream at the TV), "Put them on a real bike!" I mean, does it look like they're having a good time? At all? No. It looks like a chore they have to suffer through until the trainer says they can stop, which is pretty much how I (or any cyclist I know) feel when I'm forced to pedal aimlessly on a bike to nowhere. Sure, they may lose a few pounds churning away inside the walls of the club. But the real benefits of being on a bike—being outdoors, having fun, feeling like a kid, and truly enjoying yourself—never come across. That's a crime.

Bicycling isn't just a pleasure. It really is one of the best exercises for weight loss. It doesn't matter how much you have to lose; you can start riding a bike and travel pretty far right out of the gate. It's gentle on your joints; easy to do with your friends and family; and burns literally thousands of calories without boring you stiff (hello, stairclimber) or making you suffer (good-bye, stairclimber). It gets you out of the mind-numbing, mirrored walls of the gym and lets you instantly regain that sense of childhood freedom. It doesn't pound your knees with endless pavement like running. And, done right, it can burn fat faster.

If you've already found cycling, fantastic. You're already hooked on the benefits. Still have some weight to lose? No problem. It's possible you're just making a few common mistakes that are stalling your progress. In this book you'll find out all the facts on fat loss, including how to eat like a pro and use your bike as the ultimate weight-loss tool, and discover detailed training plans to help you lose 10, 20, 50, even 100 pounds.

There's never been a better time to take up cycling. Bikes are better (and less expensive) than they've ever been. There are more cyclists taking up the sport every day. Since 2005, the number of bike commuters has increased 36 percent, according to US Census statistics. In 1 year alone (from 2007 to 2008) the number of frequent cyclists, those riding at least twice a week, also shot up 36 percent, according to the National Sporting Goods Association. That's great news for riders because there's strength in numbers, and of course more people to ride with. But it's also great for our collective health as well as that of our planet. Scientists have recently calculated that if all Americans between the ages of 10 and 74 replaced just 30 minutes a day of traveling by car with a half hour of riding a bike, we could shed 6.5 billion pounds, save 26.1 million gallons of gasoline, and cut 255 million tons of CO_2 greenhouse gas emissions in just 1 year.

Even more important perhaps than helping you get healthy and lean in the short term, cycling will help you stay lean for life. Unlike more punishing forms of exercise, cycling is something you can do well into your sixties, seventies, and beyond. Once you've gotten down to fighting weight, this book will give you all the tools you need to stay there.

That's it. No restrictive, soul-sucking diet. No laborious, boring treadmill workouts. No punishing joint pain. Just go out, ride, and be happy. The pounds will melt away. That's our promise. Now get ready to roll.

1: THE FACTS ON FAT

WHY WE GAIN WEIGHT SO EASILY AND HOW TO LOSE IT THE SAME WAY

FACT: ACCORDING TO the surgeon general, the average American adult gains 1 to 3 pounds per year. Think about that for a second. That means if you weighed 150 pounds after graduation, you'll weigh anywhere from 170 to 210 by your 20th reunion, and even more 10 or 20 years later. But it happens so slowly (really, 0.16 pound a month—how would you notice?) that you feel like you wake up one morning reaching for anything with an elastic waistband because you have nothing left that fits.

That was how Phyllis Ingram, 63, from Barto, Pennsylvania, felt. She'd spent her adult life raising a family and tending to the needs of others. She'd always been active, riding horses and pursuing outdoor hobbies, but the time for those things shrank as her kids grew. And as her kids grew, so did she, in ways that didn't make her very happy. By age 52, she was carrying 225 pounds on her 5'6" frame. "Just walking to the second floor in my house left me winded. My knees hurt. My hips hurt. Everything hurt," she recalls. "One day I decided enough was enough. I was too young to feel so old. The weight had to go." She signed up for Spinning classes. Inspired by how fit and strong she felt pedaling in class, she bought a bike and started riding in small, casual groups. Today she is 70 pounds lighter and literally half her previous size, having dropped from a size 24 to a 12. She rides everywhere, and with her kids now grown she can take the time for some long rides, up to 100 miles on the weekends. She even started racing—and winning. "The physical benefits have been tremendous, but the mental ones are even better. I feel so much happier and more energetic. I get grumpy if I can't ride."

Maybe like Brian Strauser, 35, from Allentown, Pennsylvania, and millions of other Americans, weight has been a lifelong battle that you've been waging for as long as you can remember, and that you'd like to win once and for all. "I was always the big kid growing up. I kept my weight more or less in check by skateboarding and riding BMX. But when I graduated from high school and decided it was time to give that stuff up and be an 'adult,' the weight just started packing on. By the time I was 24 years old, I was 328 pounds. It was horrible." For Brian, it took rediscovering a childhood passion to help him get in the best shape of his life. In a single year, just riding when he could, he worked his way down to 235 pounds. He was even inspired enough to recently train for and run his first marathon. He did it, through searing knee pain, and hopped right back on his bike. Today, at around 200 pounds, he's a devoted cyclist. "There's just nothing like riding. I'll probably always have a bit of a battle with my weight. But I know my bike can help me stay on the winning side of that war."

Maybe you only have 15 pounds to lose, or 30, but I'll bet you can relate to Brian, Phyllis, and all the other now lean and happy cyclists you're going to meet in the pages of this book. If you have this book in your hands, chances are you, like them, are all too familiar with fighting fat. On paper it sounds really easy: Just eat less and move more and the pounds will peel off. Yeah, right. If it were that easy, nobody would be overweight. Anyone who has ever gained, lost, and regained (maybe multiple times) knows that it's not such a simple equation. That's why weight cycling (the lose/gain loop) is so common. The good news is that, as Phyllis and Brian have learned, bicycling can help you break the cycle and get lean for life.

✳FEAST, FAMINE, AND FAT BURN

To understand how to shed fat, it helps to understand how and why we store it in the first place. The "why" part is actually pretty simple to answer. We store fat so we have energy to burn when there's no food. The problem, which really isn't a problem when you consider the alternative, is that most of us have much more food than we really need. In fact, we now live in an environment rife with calorie pollution and with mega-conglomerates pouring millions of marketing dollars into convincing us we need to eat more. This isn't going to be a dissertation on the politics of food supply and free market capitalism, but it sure helps to know what you're up against so that you can make informed choices along the way to losing weight for good.

There are now 3,900 calories (that's about 2 days' worth for many of us) available every day to every man, woman, and child in the country, according to surveys of the US per capita food supply. No one is putting a gun to your head and forcing you to eat them, of course. But let's face it. They're everywhere and they're really tempting. From potato chips to cheesy subs to honey buns and soft pretzels, there is cheap, accessible, often delicious food available at every gas station, convenience store, concession stand, ball game, concert, and, of course, supermarket. Restaurant and packaged food portion sizes have grown to monumental proportions. We have come to associate food with entertainment; in fact, the food itself is often the main entertainment. It is very, very difficult not to eat more than planned on a daily basis. So it should come as no surprise that we are eating more—a lot more—these days. Though it's the subject of considerable debate, some experts estimate that today we eat at least 300 calories—basically an additional lunch—more each day than we did just 25 years ago. Even those who don't agree that we're consuming that much more are in complete agreement that we are burning far less, which brings us to the next point.

Each pound of body weight represents 3,500 calories of unused, stocked away, and ready-to-use energy in your body. It doesn't take a degree in mathematics to see that the excess we're taking in adds up quickly. Unless you're doing something to convert those calories into energy and burn them off, they get stored as fat molecules in your storage cells. Your body uses these fat storage cells like a savings account, in case you need energy when food is scarce. As you've likely noticed, this is a pretty efficient system. For most of us, it's far easier to "pad" our biological savings account than it is to empty it out.

In theory, it should be easy. You've likely heard a million times that weight loss is simply a matter of calories in versus calories out. So if you just burn 500 more calories than you eat, you should tap into your fat storage cells and lose about a pound a week. Were it only that simple. Like everything else in weight loss, fat burning is not such a perfect equation. Even the most respected exercise physiologists in the world confess that scientists still know woefully little about how we actually burn calories. Why else would universities around the globe conduct hundreds of studies each year trying to understand how exercise and diet create weight loss?

"The problem is that we're not perfect engines who process and burn energy identically," explains Tim Church, MD, PhD, MPH, professor at Pennington Biomedical Research Center at Louisiana State University System in Baton Rouge. We are individual human beings who are ruled by our own unique biology. Just look around your close circle of family and friends. It's no secret that some people can eat with abandon without gaining an ounce, while others gain weight at the slightest indulgence. The way we burn, use, and store energy is determined by a host of factors, including metabolism, body composition, and genetics. People who burn a lot of fat during the day have a tendency to send calories to short-term storage within their muscles, so they have easy access for energy to burn, explains Dr. Church. Others are more like squirrels, stashing calories for long-term storage in fat tissue. This fuel partitioning is partly genetic. But it's not immutable. Genetics, as they say, loads the gun, but lifestyle goes a long way in pulling the trigger. This is where exercise, specifically cycling, comes in, because it is one of the easiest ways to turn your body into a better fat burner.

Within each of us is an intricate system of hormones and enzymes, including insulin (well known for its role in regulating blood sugar) and lipoprotein lipase (LPL), whose job it is to make sure that fuel goes to the right places for burning and storage. Then there's your circulatory system, whose job it is to deliver all these hormones and nutrient-rich blood to their proper places. Well, guess what? Your lifestyle and exercise habits can have a tremendous impact on these systems, both positively and negatively. On the negative side, being sedentary for too long sends all these systems into hibernation. New "inactivity research" (a brand-new body of science based on our depressingly sedentary lives) shows that when you sit for a few hours, your body literally starts to shut down on the metabolic level. Fat-burning enzymes like LPL begin switching off. Sit at your desk (or on the sofa) for a full day, and LPL activity plummets by 50 percent. It's a slippery slope downhill from here. Unless you get up and get moving, your body goes deeper into energy-conservation mode. Your circulation slows. Your digestion becomes sluggish. Your calorie-burning furnaces cool to a flicker. Thanks to the computerization of everything from online banking to shopping to, now, even socializing, we sit more than any people have in the history of mankind. As a result experts estimate that today we burn 1,000 fewer calories—that's half a day's worth—per day than we did just 30 years ago.

Moving more is obviously the answer. And, as you'll soon discover, cycling is the perfect exercise whether you have a little weight to lose or a lot.

PEDAL POWER

What makes cycling so special for weight loss? Let's start with the mechanics. Bicycling is a nonimpact exercise, which means there's no jarring on your joints, so even the heaviest rider can climb aboard a bike and pedal. With today's fully geared bicycles, anyone from the most out-of-shape beginner to the recreational racer can pedal in comfort for miles. Cycling also uses all the biggest muscles in your body—your quads, hamstrings, hip muscles, and glutes. That's all essential for improving your fat-burning ability.

Cycling, especially long, steady rides, builds hundreds of thousands of capillaries in your legs, which means you can deliver more oxygen-rich blood to your working muscles. At the same time, your mitochondria—the fat-burning furnaces in your muscle cells—get bigger, so they can use the increased influx of oxygen to burn more fat and produce more energy. In one study of relatively sedentary men and women, after just 8 weeks of riding five times a week for 30 minutes, they increased their capillary-per-fiber ratio (a fancy way of saying how many blood vessels per muscle fiber) in their quads by 40 percent, the density of their mitochondria by 15 percent, and the amount of oxygen their legs could use during exercise by nearly as much (13 percent). All that after just 2 months. In another study, researchers found that bicyclists' LPL (fat-burning enzyme) activity was elevated for a full 30 hours after riding. The kind of endurance training you do on a bicycle also elevates your levels of fatty-acid-binding proteins and fat-carrying enzymes so your body is more efficient at shuttling fatty acids from storage into your working muscles. Simply put, the fitter you get, the more oxygen you can use, and the more fat you can burn.

Cycling also increases your daily calorie burn. First, and most obviously, cycling burns calories—hundreds of them—while you're out there turning the pedals. Even at a recreational pace of 13 to 15 miles per hour, you burn 500 to 600 calories in 1 hour or about 4,000 per week—enough to burn off more than a pound—if you ride just an hour every day. Cycling also coaxes your body to continue burning calories at a higher rate after you've racked your bike, because your body is still working to repair and replenish your muscles. Finally, bicycling builds lean muscle tissue and raises your basal metabolic rate (BMR), the calories you burn while you're just hanging around, not exercising. Studies show that just 30 to 45 minutes of exercise most days a week can boost your BMR and keep it raised. As if that weren't enough, most people find cycling so energizing that they're simply more active, and hence burning more calories, all day long.

Though you can't "spot-reduce"—that is, lose body fat in any one particular trouble spot—you can through cycling build lean muscle tissue in your lower body and trim fat from around your middle. In fact, even before you see a single pound disappear from the scale, cycling begins melting away deep, dangerous belly fat from your middle. In one study of 24 men and women with diabetes, ages 45 and older, those who biked 45 minutes three times a week for 8 weeks decreased their visceral fat (the deep belly fat that smothers your organs and leads to heart disease, diabetes, and other disease) by 48 percent.

While we're talking about fat burning and loss, ignore what you might hear about "the fat-burning zone." You'll find a complete discussion of this in Chapter 3, but suffice it to say that while you do technically burn more fat at lower riding intensities, you still burn plenty of fat when you ride briskly or even vigorously, and you burn more calories too. In a study at Georgia State University, researchers found that riders doing either short, hard rides or longer, more mellow rides of equal calorie burn shed the same amount of fat regardless of riding intensity. But don't worry. The plans in Chapter 4 will do all the strategizing for you. All you have to do is ride.

✳ SNEAKY WAYS CYCLING TAKES OFF POUNDS

Calorie burning and muscle building are the obvious ways cycling helps you drop unwanted pounds. But that's just the beginning. Here are a few stealth and sometimes surprising ways that bicycling can help you shed body fat fast.

Bicycling makes you happy. A recent study from Bowling Green State University reported that as little as 10 minutes of cycling improved the mood among 21 men and women, compared to a similar group who did nothing during that time. Other research shows that just 30 minutes of aerobic activity, like cycling, per day 3 to 5 days a week can significantly improve depression symptoms, and that more brisk activities like bicycling may work even faster.

Feeling happier can help you beat fat by reducing the likelihood that you'll reach for a mood boost in a pint of ice cream or plow your way through a pizza to burn off the blues after a bad day at work. Cornell University researchers have found that people who are sad tend to not only eat more food but also eat more high-carbohydrate, high-calorie comfort food than those who feel happy.

Bicycling gives you more energy to burn. Funny story: The other day I rode over to meet my husband for a lunchtime ride by Lehigh University, where he works. I arrived at the parking lot to see a line of cars, all their owners sitting with their front seats pushed back, napping in sunny parking spots. "That used to be me," I thought with a smile. Years prior, I was working in New Jersey, and I'd fallen out of the habit of riding, running, or pretty much doing anything. I'd sit at my desk from 8:30 to noon, some days barely able to keep my eyes open. Come lunchtime, I (and several of my co-workers) would go to our cars, park them in sunny spots, and take naps before parking ourselves back at our computers for the remainder of the day, struggling to keep our eyelids from falling from 3 p.m. on. The malaise of the day would follow me home, as I'd half-heartedly make dinner and plop myself in front of the TV until bedtime. I grew soft and sad.

Then I discovered people who ran and rode bikes at lunchtime. I wasn't sure how they had the energy to do so, but I wanted to be one of them. The results were both amazing and instantaneous. The day I decided to ride at lunch, I was excited (and nervous) all morning. No thoughts of napping. No nodding off. Though it was a little tough getting the sluggish legs moving at first, once we were going, the ride was awesome. We chatted and laughed, pushed hard up hills, and coasted down them. I returned to work completely invigorated and far more productive than I'd ever been post parking lot snooze. It's a lesson that stuck. Energy begets energy. The more you move, the more you'll want to move. And it's not just me talking. It's thousands of people and some hard science.

When University of Georgia researchers analyzed data from 70 studies on exercise and fatigue that involved more than 6,800 men and women, they found that 90 percent of the studies reported the same result: Exercise increases energy and reduces fatigue. Sedentary people who participated in an exercise program experienced less fatigue than their still-sedentary counterparts, and the average energy boost was actually greater than improvements reported from using stimulant medications. The energy boost was similar for nearly every group, healthy to chronically ill, including people who had heart disease, cancer, and diabetes. Tired of being tired? Get a bike.

Bicycling leads to better sleep. Because it gives you so much energy during the day, bicycling will help you sleep like a baby during the night, which is a very good thing when you consider the sorry state of most of our nights of shut-eye. Sleep statistics show that the average night's sleep has dropped from 9 hours to 7 during the past 20 years, with many of us getting a whole lot less. That's bad news for your weight-loss efforts, say scientists, because when you don't give your body the sleep it craves, it starts hunting for relief in the form of food.

Remember how pulling all-nighters in college was easier when you had a bag of chips to keep you company? That's because when you're tired, your body pumps out higher levels of a key appetite-regulating hormone called ghrelin, which makes you feel hungry and helps keep you alert. Worse, you won't be reaching for an apple and a glass of milk to quell the cravings. You'll be more apt to fill up on sugary foods to boost your blood sugar and charge your energy levels. Interestingly, researchers find that even men and women who ate less during periods of low sleep still gained weight, likely because their bodies were slipping into energy-conservation mode and they were not burning calories as efficiently.

The statistics on sleep and weight are startling. The Nurses' Health Study, which studied the sleep habits and body weight trends among more than 68,000 women for more than 16 years, found that those who slept only 5 hours a night were 32 percent more likely to gain 33 pounds or more over the course of the study, and were 15 percent more likely to become obese than those who slept 7 hours a night. There was even a pronounced difference among those who slept 6 hours a night (12 percent more likely to experience major weight gain) than those who got 7.

Regular bicycling can help you fall asleep faster, sleep more soundly, and get more overall shut-eye. When Stanford University researchers asked 43 men and women with mild sleep troubles to do 30 to 40 minutes of aerobic exercise, which included bike riding, 4 days a week, they found that after 16 weeks the volunteers were able to fall asleep about 15 minutes faster and slept about 45 minutes longer each night. That's a full hour of extra sleep from very little exercise.

How daily exercise lulls you into easy nighttime slumber is still not completely understood, but researchers believe it's a combination of reducing stress and regulating your circadian rhythms. Bicycling also gets you out in the fresh air and sunshine, both of which have been shown to improve biological rhythms as well.

Bicycling blunts your appetite. Here's a controversial one. Many people who are trying to cut calories and lose weight worry that exercising will make them eat more. For some people, that's true, particularly if they turn to food as a reward for working out. But in terms of real appetite, the evidence indicates that the opposite is true. Studies of overweight men and women who start exercising show that vigorous exercise actually suppresses appetite for a few hours afterward. Likewise, Tufts University researchers reported in a review article that people generally enjoy a "spontaneous reduction in hunger" when they start exercising, which they noted also consistently led to weight loss.

Aerobic exercise, like bicycling, seems to blunt appetite on more than one level. First, bicycling raises your dopamine levels and lights up the pleasure centers of your brain. It simply makes you feel good, supplanting the need for other mood boosters like chips and salsa or chocolate chip cookies. Second, researchers from Loughborough University in the United Kingdom have reported that 60 minutes of vigorous exercise, like brisk bicycling, lowers the release of ghrelin, a hormone that stimulates appetite, and increases the release of peptide YY, a hormone that suppresses appetite.

Bicycling relieves stress. Though scientists are still unraveling the biological facts, there appears to be a direct connection between unchecked stress and weight gain. It comes down to what we've come to know as our fight-or-flight response. When you're under stress, whether at home or work, or maybe unfortunately both, your body goes into fight-or-flight mode, physically preparing you to either knock someone's lights out or run like heck. Your heart beats faster and harder. Your cells pump fatty acids into your bloodstream to fuel your muscles. And your adrenal glands amp their production of stress hormones like cortisol to put your whole body on high alert and ready for action. Chances are, however, you are going to start neither swinging nor sprinting, but are more likely to sit stewing in this toxic pool of high stress.

This resignation in the face of stress creates its own metabolic cascade of events that leads to increased fat production, especially in the belly, where it does the most damage, as well as suppressed immunity. It also sends many men and women to the fridge, vending machine, or convenience store for a quick feel-better food fix. By exercising, you give your body a healthy outlet for pent-up stress. Aerobic exercise like pedaling a bike uses up excess adrenaline and slows the production of cortisol. It also stimulates endorphins and other good-mood chemicals that lower your anxiety and improve your sense of well-being.

Bicycling is fun. When people want to know the "best" exercise for weight loss, experts universally agree that it's the one you enjoy. And bicycling is highly enjoyable. But don't just take our word for it. Take Mark Blaubach's. Mark, of Kerrville, Texas, lost 117 pounds (he started at 364) after buying a mountain bike when his doctor ordered him to lose weight or end up in the morgue. "Burning calories has to be fun! If it feels too much like work, you'll eventually find an excuse *not* to do it. I tried everything. And everything felt like drudgery . . . until I bought a bike. It sounds cliché, but I felt like a kid again. It was still hard exercise. At first I had to push my bike up the smallest of hills. But it didn't feel like work. It's the love of bicycling that has enabled me to keep the weight off for over 10 years," says Mark, now 41, whose wife, Faye, got the biking bug shortly thereafter and found herself 50 pounds lighter. "That was 10 years ago, and we've been happily biking away ever since," Mark says with a smile.

Bicycling makes you healthier. A healthy body simply functions better, allowing you to live more fully and, of course, burn more calories in the process. For John Turney, 63, of Concord, California, riding was practically doctor's orders. "In August 2008, I went to my cardiologist for a routine visit, and my blood pressure was measured as high. I had been really glued to my desk for the past couple of years, and my back was starting to hurt. And at 6'0", I weighed 218 pounds. The doctor prescribed weight loss for everything." John cut back on his portions and started to jog. It worked and the weight was coming off until his knees said, "No more," just 8 months later. "The doctor told me not to jog. I had never been athletic, so we discussed my options. Swimming (I'm terrible), treadmills (how boring), and cycling. He and I convinced my wife that cycling was the way to go. On the way home we stopped by REI to buy her a water bottle, and I bought a hybrid bike." Just like that, John fell in love with riding.

In 6 months, he put 1,500 miles on the hybrid and kept losing weight and getting fitter and faster. He also started weight-training 2 days a week. "The nice thing about riding and weight training is I can eat more (but not too much) again and the weight loss is all fat and not muscle." Inspired by his progress and ready to take his riding to another level, John just bought a Fuji road bike. Today, he's down to a healthy, pain-free 171 pounds, which makes him and his doctor happy. "I go for nice long rides before big meals (like Thanksgiving dinner), so I can keep the weight off. Last Saturday I told the fellow who runs the gym where I work out that I was going for a ride to train for Sunday. He asked if I was racing. I said, 'No, I have an all-you-can-eat champagne brunch.' I look and feel younger. It's a nice thing."

✳KEEPING IT OFF

Losing a lot of weight is sort of like climbing Everest. With the right help and strategy, almost anyone can get up the mountain. But once you reach the summit, you're only halfway there—you have to get back down, or for someone who wants to lose weight, maintain your weight loss. Surveys show that people who lose a significant amount of weight end up eventually regaining some of it, with many regaining all of it or even more. The one common factor among those who successfully keep lost pounds gone for good: exercise and plenty of it.

According to the National Weight Control Registry, which is a nearly decade-old project devoted to studying 3,500 men and women who have lost (and kept off) 60 pounds or more, one of the key indicators of long-term weight-loss success is a high weekly calorie burn. On average, women who have successfully lost and maintained big weight loss burn 2,545 calories a week; their male peers burn 3,293. Similar research has reported that the magic calorie-burn number for weight loss and maintenance is about 2,000 calories or 4.5 to 5 hours of moderate exercise a week—that's about twice the typical recommendation of 30 minutes of exercise most days a week—but very easy (as you'll soon see) to do on a bike.

Burning calories is the obvious way that exercise keeps weight at bay. But there's more to the slimming effects than meets the eye. A University of Colorado Denver study found that exercise helps prevent weight regain on a number of fronts. Most interestingly, it seems to metabolically reset your body's "defended weight," or the default weight your body tries to maintain through appetite and fat storage. It also prevents your body from adding fat cells (more cells mean more capacity for storage) during the "relapse" period when dieters are no longer following a strict regimen. Regular exercise also appears to reduce the urge to overeat and enhances your body's ability to balance energy intake with energy expended. The end result: less weight regain.

But that's just all the science speak. More important in the whole yo-yo diet discussion, cycling gets you off the treadmill—literally. It gets you away from the dull, pointless chore of "exercise" (i.e., elliptical machine) and makes you feel carefree and like a kid again. A long, challenging ride fills you with a sense of accomplishment and joy that lingers long after you've showered up and gone back to the rigors of daily living. Bicycling is something you can do forever, long after you may have hung up your running shoes or simply grown weary of schlepping to the gym. Research shows that positive mood and consistent activity both go an awful long way in weight maintenance, which is certainly not rocket science.

A bicycle is simply the perfect vehicle for shedding pounds and keeping them off. It's easy to rack up a big calorie burn; it's fun to do; you can do it with friends and family; you can fit it in your everyday life to run errands around town; and you can pedal well into your old age, even when aches and pains make it tough to walk.

✳MAGIC NUMBERS: WEIGHT, BMI, WAISTLINE—WHAT MATTERS MOST

When I ask clients what their goals are, weight loss is inevitably high on the list. That's not surprising, of course. What is surprising is the random, magical, nearly mythical numbers they pull out when they tell me what they would like to weigh. It's always very specific, like 185 or 130, a weight they think they "should" weigh. Sometimes it's incredibly precise, like 128 or 163, numbers I call "happy time weight," which is usually what they weighed during a time when everything was going swimmingly well, like their senior year of high school, or when they got married.

Most of us have these magic numbers. But they're not always realistic or even ideal. Further, the numbers on the scale are only one piece of the fitness puzzle. The complete picture is revealed by your body type, body composition, BMI, and for cycling success, your power-to-weight ratio. Here's a look at how the measurements measure up and what it all means for you.

What's Your Build?

Most people have a pretty good sense of their general build, or overall body type. Whether you are muscular or wiry, big boned (as your grandmother might say) or petite helps determine your healthy weight. That's why there's a 35-pound difference between the lowest and the highest healthy weights for any given height. A small-framed 5'10" man is perfectly healthy carrying 150 pounds, but might be overweight at 175, which would be the ideal weight for a man of the same height with a larger stature. The same is true for a 5'4" woman, who could weigh anywhere from 114 to 151 and still be considered a healthy weight depending on her frame size.

Just as mountain bike manufacturers generally offer their bikes in S, M, L, depending on frame dimensions, insurance companies typically divide weight categories into small-, medium-, and large-frame categories. Just as you whip out a measuring tape to check a bike's dimensions, you can check your own frame size with a simple measurement: the distance between the two little bones on either side of your elbow.

Hold your arm at a 90-degree angle with your palm facing yourself. With your other hand feel the two bones that make up your elbow joint. Put your index finger on one of the bones and your thumb on the other. Then measure the distance between them. Use the chart below to determine your frame size. The measurements here are for a medium-size frame. If your measurements are lower for your height, you have a small frame; if they're higher for your height, your frame is large.

medium-frame measurements

HEIGHT	ELBOW BREADTH
5'2" and under	2.25"–2.5"
5'3"–5'10"	2.375"–2.625"
5'11" and up	2.5"–2.75"

Once you know your frame size, consider your general build. Going back to the bike frame analogy, you'll notice that some frames are thick, some are thin, and others fall somewhere in between. People, too, tend to be a wide variety of builds, with most of us being either ectomorphs, who tend to be long limbed and not particularly muscular; mesomorphs, who are generally very muscular; and endomorphs, who tend to be more heavy set. Muscle tissue is dense, so someone with a lot of muscle is always going to be heavier than someone with less. That's why it's important to not wrap your fitness goals tightly around a magical number you weighed when you were 19. Even if you lose all your unwanted fat, you may simply have more muscle now (a good thing!), so you'll weigh more no matter what you do.

Shown opposite are healthy weight ranges for men and women, according to the Metropolitan Life Insurance Company tables (1983).

weight chart for women

HEIGHT	SMALL FRAME	MEDIUM FRAME	LARGE FRAME
4'10"	102–111	109–121	118–131
4'11"	103–113	111–123	120–134
5'0"	104–115	113–126	122–137
5'1"	106–118	115–129	125–140
5'2"	108–121	118–132	128–143
5'3"	111–124	121–135	131–147
5'4"	114–127	124–138	134–151
5'5"	117–130	127–141	137–155
5'6"	120–133	130–144	140–159
5'7"	123–136	133–147	143–163
5'8"	126–139	136–150	146–167
5'9"	129–142	139–153	149–170
5'10"	132–145	142–156	152–173
5'11"	135–148	145–159	155–176
6'0"	138–151	148–162	158–179

weight chart for men

HEIGHT	SMALL FRAME	MEDIUM FRAME	LARGE FRAME
5'2"	128–134	131–141	138–150
5'3"	130–136	133–143	140–153
5'4"	132–138	135–145	142–156
5'5"	134–140	137–148	144–160
5'6"	136–142	139–151	146–164
5'7"	138–145	142–154	149–168
5'8"	140–148	145–157	152–172
5'9"	142–151	148–160	155–176
5'10"	144–154	151–163	158–180
5'11"	146–157	154–166	161–184
6'0"	149–160	157–170	164–188
6'1"	152–164	160–174	168–192
6'2"	155–168	164–178	172–197
6'3"	158–172	167–182	176–202
6'4"	162–176	171–187	181–207

BMI

Body mass index (BMI) became all the rage in the nineties as a better tool for measuring body composition. It's basically a height/weight formula that figures out how much of you there is in every square inch of your body. As a ballpark figure, it works fairly well. But it has definite limitations for active, muscular people, because, as mentioned earlier, muscle tissue is dense and heavier than other tissues, especially fat. So if you're very muscular, your BMI can easily (and erroneously) slip into the overweight category. Using BMI as a guide, most football players, for instance, would be considered obese.

Still, it can be a good number to know, and for many people it can be a good indicator of their general health, since myriad weight-associated health woes such as heart disease, diabetes, and even some cancers can be linked to having a too-high BMI. You can figure out your BMI yourself using a complex mathematical formula. But it's far easier to use one of the many BMI calculators available on the Internet, like this one from the Centers for Disease Control and Prevention found at the following link: www.cdc.gov/healthyweight/assessing/bmi/.

This chart tells you what your number means.

BMI	WEIGHT STATUS
Below 18.5	Underweight
18.5—24.9	Normal
25.0—29.9	Overweight
30.0 and above	Obese

Waistline

More important than how much fat you have in your body is where that fat sits. You've likely heard that some people are apples, meaning they wear their excess pounds around their middle, while others are pears, those who tend to deposit extra pounds below the belt. (There are others, of course, who have their weight pretty evenly distributed.) This impacts more than your physical profile. Scientists now know that people who tend to carry fat around their waist have more visceral fat, which is located deep inside the abdominal cavity. This deep fat surrounds the internal organs. Unlike subcutaneous fat (the kind that sits directly beneath the skin), which hangs out in storage waiting to be burned, visceral fat tends to be more metabolically active, acting almost like its own organ, pumping out hormones, fatty acids, and other substances that can harm your health.

This chemical cavalcade can pave the way for chronic diseases of all kinds, especially diabetes, high blood pressure, high cholesterol, atherosclerosis, heart disease, and even hormone-fueled cancers like those of the breast, colon, and prostate. Even people with moderate amounts of weight to lose can have excessive amounts of abdominal fat, which is why waist circumference has become the go-to measurement of choice for many doctors trying to get a snapshot of overall health risk. It's also a better measurement than BMI for people who are classified as overweight only because they are heavily muscular.

That's the bad news. The good news is that your body tends to dig into your deep fat stores first when you start exercising to lose weight, so you'll be tightening your belt and improving your health almost immediately after you start to ride, and it'll just improve with each pedal stroke.

To determine your waist circumference, find the top of your hip bones on either side of your body. Place the measuring tape around your waist at this point so it wraps around your waist parallel to the floor. Breathe normally (don't suck in your stomach) and hold the tape taut, but not tight; it should not cut into your skin. According to the US Department of Health and Human Services, you're at an increased risk for the diseases just mentioned when your waistline measures more than 40 inches if you're a man or more than 35 inches if you're a woman. But don't get too discouraged if you have a long way to go to bring your belt into that territory. According to weight-loss research, trimming just 2¼ inches off your waistline can reduce your cholesterol 9 percent, your triglycerides by 26 percent, and blood pressure 8 percent.

Body Composition

BMI and waist circumference are good ballpark gauges of your body composition. But the only way to really know what you're made of, so to speak, is to get a body composition test, which breaks down your weight into percent fat and lean tissue.

There are many methods of determining body composition. The two most commonly available are bioelectrical impedance analysis (BIA) and skinfold measurement. BIA works by sending electrical signals (don't worry, you can't feel them) through your body. These signals react differently as they pass through fat, lean mass, and water. So based on how the currents react, the machine calculates your body composition percentages. You can even buy BIA scales for home use. When done properly, BIA is pretty accurate. But hydration levels, food intake, exercise, skin temperature, and other factors can skew the readings, so it's important to follow the directions to the letter for the best results. Skinfold measurement is done by using special calipers to gently pinch the fat beneath the skin at various sites on your body, like the triceps, hip, back, and thigh. It, too, is very accurate—up to 98 percent accurate, according to the American College of Sports Medicine—if done correctly, though it's important that the person doing the measuring is well trained.

The nice thing about having body composition readings is you can watch the magic of cycling at work in ways that a scale alone can't show. As you ride, you build lean muscle tissue, especially in your legs and glutes, while you're shedding fat from all over. Muscle takes up less space than fat, but it weighs more, so even though your fat stores are shrinking, you may not see a big absolute weight change right away. You will, however, see a body composition change, which can be pretty satisfying.

The numbers you're shooting for vary depending on your gender, since women naturally have more body fat than men. You need a certain amount of fat to live, so you're not gunning for zero. The body fat ranges for optimal health are 18 to 30 percent for women and 10 to 25 percent for men. Body fat percentages for fitness are obviously a bit lower than those for general good health, as the chart (opposite) shows.

	WOMEN (%)	MEN (%)
Essential fat	Less than 8	Less than 5
Athletes	12–22	5–13
General fitness	16–25	12–18
Good health	18–30	10–25
Too high	Over 30	Over 25

POWER-TO-WEIGHT RATIO

Of all the measurements, this one's my favorite, because it's most meaningful to you, the cyclist. As the name implies, it's the amount of power, measured in watts, that you can generate per kilogram (kg), or 2.2 pounds, of body weight. You need a power meter (a special wattage-reading meter) on your bike to actually measure your power to weight. You find the number by riding as hard as you can for 20 to 30 minutes (the best way to do this is on a long climb) and determining your average power output. Then divide your weight in kilograms into that number. So if you weigh 180 pounds (82 kg) and you averaged 275 watts, your power-to-weight ratio would be 3.4 watts/kg. What does that mean? For reference, top Tour de France racers boast power-to-weight ratios of 6.8 watts/kg. Beginner cyclists usually pull in the range of 2.5 to 3.2 for men and 2.1 to 2.8 for women. Fast recreational riders crank out wattage in the range of 3.7 to 4.4 for men and 3.2 to 3.8 for women.

As you may have already guessed, you can improve your power to weight two ways: drop weight and get stronger. As you continue riding, you'll find that you'll be doing both. There are also specific power-building drills in later chapters to give you an even bigger boost. Improving your power-to-weight ratio is good for more than an ego boost. It helps you motor up hard hills and actually enjoy climbing as opposed to suffering up every incline. That's why guys who may actually look scrawny can often fly up the mountains as if powered by wings. They have to generate less power to push their weight against the pull of gravity. Top-notch climbers generally have less than 2 pounds of body weight per inch of height. So if you were 5'10", you'd weigh about 140 pounds. But don't worry! We're not looking to qualify for the Olympics here, but rather to lose some weight and enjoy the ride.

2:GEARING UP FOR THE ROAD TO WEIGHT LOSS

FROM YOUR BIKE TO YOUR BUTT—
EVERYTHING YOU NEED FOR YOUR CYCLING
PLEASURE

IF YOU KNEW cycling only through the lens of a Tour de France camera, you would conclude that it's a skinny man's sport. There are no linebackers in the pro peloton. That is true. But outside of the professional ranks there are plenty of Clydesdales and Athenas (larger male and female cyclists) happily pedaling along. As a bigger rider, however, you (and your behind . . . and your wallet) will be even happier if you choose the right gear.

"When I slung my leg over my first mountain bike, I was over 300 pounds," recalls Brian Strauser. "At that time, clothing companies didn't make cycling clothes for guys as big as me. The equipment also didn't hold up so well. My first bike was a GT Saddleback I bought for $289 at Nestor's. I destroyed the rims right away. I also bottomed out the cheap front shock absorber. I even bent seatposts. I was embarrassed to even head into the woods looking like I did on top of my bike and breaking things. But I learned a ton; it saved my life, and I would do it all again!"

Phyllis Ingram didn't break anything, but finding clothing that fit was nearly futile. "There were no flattering clothes. I had to buy men's XL cycling shorts, jerseys, and jackets," says Phyllis. Fortunately, those days are in the past as more and more cycling manufacturers recognize that millions of people, including plus-size people, are getting on bikes and want quality merchandise so they can look good, feel good, and, in the case of bikes, be safe doing it. Here we'll help you gear up with exactly what you need.

❋WHEN LIGHT IS TOO LIGHT

When considering what bike to buy, one of your top considerations should be weight—not just yours, but the bike's and its parts'. Cyclists tend to get caught up in weight, measuring everything down to their pedals to the nearest gram. That's fine if you have a pro contract or you're a flyweight Spanish climber who has to belt his size zero True Religion jeans. But ultralight components don't always make sense for most everyday riders, especially those who are heavier. For one, they're very expensive. More important, they don't hold up. A very big rider can potentially taco (read: bend in half, like a taco shell) ultralight wheels or even snap pro-level stems and seatposts (those oh-so-important parts that attach your handlebars and your seat to your bike). So it's pretty important that larger riders gravitate toward components that can bear their weight. And in the world of cycling, heavyweight ain't all that heavy. A rider who weighs more than 180 pounds will actually void the warranty of some very high-end products, such as certain titanium pedals, saddles with carbon fiber rails, and lightweight carbon handlebars and stems.

That all may sound a bit elitist, and honestly, it may be a little bit, since there's some snobbery at the top ranks of any sport. But there's also a matter of practicality. In this power-to-weight sport, the riders who are as light as birds are looking to buy power through featherweight components. Most of the extremely low-weight, high-performance products are designed specifically for racing and for the skinny riders who race professionally. When you're carrying extra pounds on your personal frame, it's smarter (and far more cost effective) to drop some weight before shelling out hundreds (or more likely thousands) of dollars to shed a few ounces on your bike. That is not to say, however, that you must then relegate yourself to bargain-basement goods.

"It's really only pro-level, pure racing gear that can't support riders over 180 to 200 pounds," says *Bicycling* magazine deputy test editor Mike Cushionbury. "Most everything you buy off the floor of your local bike shop is fine for even very heavy riders. Great parts like Dura-Ace pedals, SRAM Red cranks, and Deda alloy handlebars will hold up to heavier weights." It's when you move into the 230-pound-and-beyond range that regular bike parts start to be put to their limits, he says. It also depends on what you're doing. If you're just cruising along, many products will still be fine, notes Cushionbury. But start hammering away, and it might be more wear and tear than the components can take under weight.

If you are in the 230-pound-and-beyond range, you should pay special attention to your wheels, if nothing else, notes *Bicycling* test editor Ron Koch. "The first thing to fail on bikes under extreme weights are the wheels. Heavier riders should look for wheels with aluminum rims and 36 rather than 32 spokes, because they'll hold up better."

✳MOUNTAIN, ROAD, OR IN-BETWEEN

Your first decision is what type of bike to buy. Many new riders coming into the sport looking to lose weight put their money on a mountain bike or a hybrid because they feel more stable. Take Susan Donnelly, 48, of Woonsocket, Rhode Island, who wrote to us at *Bicycling* recalling her weight-loss journey that began at 286 pounds. "At first I bought a hybrid and rode that on the trails," she recalls. "Then when I had lost 100 pounds, I purchased a road bike." She loved it so much that she and her husband decided to train to ride a century (a 100-mile bike ride). Now 130 pounds lighter, Susan is thrilled. "For the first time in my life I'm medication free. I no longer suffer from depression. I have no joint discomfort, and my chronic headaches are gone."

What type of bike you ultimately choose depends on what kind of riding you'll be doing, where you'll be doing it, and your comfort level. Of course, if you want to ride on the dirt, you should get a mountain bike, or on the road, a road bike. But even within those broad categories there are still many choices. Read on for what to consider.

Road. For those new to cycling, when you see Lance Armstrong and pro cycling on TV, you're looking at road bikes. Constructed from lightweight materials like aluminum, steel, titanium, or carbon fiber, these machines are built for speed. Curved "drop" handlebars allow you to tuck into a fast, aerodynamic position. The tires are skinny for the least amount of rolling resistance on the road.

This category is enormous, offering a wide variety of road bikes to choose from, from ultraresponsive top-shelf race bikes (which new riders may find too aggressive and unstable) to sturdier touring bikes, which may not be as nimble but take a lot of abuse and keep coming back for more. Riders who like to sit a little more upright rather than far forward are generally more comfortable on a touring or more relaxed, recreationally minded road bike than a pure performance race bike. One category all riders would be wise to consider is what *Bicycling* magazine deems a "plush" bike—a bike that is designed for comfort as well as speed. "These bikes have a taller head tube and slightly shorter top tube, so the rider sits a bit more upright. They also have vibration absorption built into the frame, so the ride isn't as rigid as a more aggressive road racing bike," explains Cushionbury. Yet, the bikes are still relatively light and the overall geometry responsive, so when you want to open it up, the bike goes fast. The Specialized Roubaix was the pioneer of the plush category. Some others to consider: Cannondale Synapse Carbon, Cervélo RS, Scott CR1, Trek Pilot, Giant Defy Advanced, Bianchi Infinito.

Mountain. For off-road riders this is the bike of choice. For those new to the sport, you'll recognize them by their very beefy tires and upright design. Mountain bikes are very specifically crafted to ride on dirt paths and mountain trails. They usually have at least one shock absorber (generally in the front) to absorb the impact from riding over rocks, roots, and bumpy terrain. The handlebars are straight and wide, so you have better steering control, and the overall position is more upright, so you can easily manipulate the bike through trees and other obstacles. Though they're built for off-road riding, you can (and many people do) use them to ride on the road. The upside of riding a mountain bike is they're very stable, so even the sketchiest beginner will feel confident behind the handlebars. The downside is they're heavier and slower on the pavement than a road-specific bike, so you won't experience the zippy feeling of riding really fast. If you plan on riding mostly off road, however, this is the bike for you.

Hybrid. A little bit road, a little bit off-road, hybrids feature medium-size tires that let you roll briskly on the pavement, yet provide stability on moderately rough terrain like dirt roads or cinder paths. The position is more upright than aero, so they make comfortable commuters and good all-around exercise bikes. Some hybrids come with flat, mountain-bike-style handlebars for those who are intimidated by traditional drop-style bars. But if you do go with a flat bar, look for one with bar-ends, or extensions at the end of the handlebars that allow another option for gripping the bar. Otherwise, you risk numb, tired hands (a somewhat common complaint among larger riders) from holding your weight in the exact same position during long rides.

Once you've decided on a bike type, go out and test-drive a few. Head to your local bike shop rather than to a big-box store like Wal-Mart. Department store bikes may seem like a bargain, but when it comes to cycling, you really do get what you pay for—and what you get off the floor at Kmart is a heavy, inferior bike that won't be much fun to ride. Your bike shop will also be your go-to source for repairs, ancillary gear, places to ride, people to ride with, and much more. If you don't get the service you expect at the first shop you enter, leave and try another. Though most shops are friendly and accommodating to riders of all shapes, sizes, and experience, you'll run across the few who seem to only give the time of day to what they deem "real cyclists." No need to give them your hard-earned cash when there are plenty of places that will give you the attention you deserve.

Be sure to take out at least three bikes so you can get a real comparison. Put them through the paces by taking them up hills, pedaling quickly, and trying to come to a quick stop (safely, of course). Pay special attention to details of each bike, like how quickly and fluidly the chain moves when you shift and how smoothly it comes to a stop when you squeeze the brakes. These are features that have a profound impact on the quality of your ride and how much you'll enjoy being out on your bike. Treat yourself to the best bike you can afford. It will pay for itself in durability, performance, and sheer enjoyment of the ride.

Finally, don't leave the shop without a bike fitting. The bike shop technician can help you adjust your handlebar and seat positioning so everything fits and feels just right. Cycling is gentle on your body, but it does require that you perform a repetitive motion (pedaling) in a relatively fixed position. So even small fit imperfections, like a seat that's too low, can cause discomfort and discourage you from riding.

✳BUT SERIOUSLY . . .

One of the top concerns riders, especially heavier riders, have is sitting their behinds on a skinny bike saddle (the technical term for bike seat). What many don't realize is that it doesn't matter how much flesh you have on your fanny; what you're actually sitting on are your sit bones, which will fit comfortably on a traditional narrow saddle, no matter how wide your actual behind is. Though you can buy an extra-wide, super-cushiony saddle, if it doesn't fit your sit bones, it may end up being less comfortable than one that is narrow and firm. Because those bones are spaced differently on everybody, the key for comfort is finding a saddle on which the rear supports those bones in the riding position. Some bike shops actually have a special device that you sit on that measures your sit-bone width. But at the least, most shops will let you try a few saddles to see which one fits you best.

When choosing your saddle, also consider the kind of riding you'll be doing. A narrower saddle is better for the kind of fast pedaling you'll be striving for to lose weight. Unlike a relaxed "beach cruiser" position that places your hands higher than your seat and your weight back onto your rear (hence creating a need for a wider, more fully supportive saddle), a fitness riding position places your weight forward so it is evenly distributed on your hands and feet and butt, which reduces the total weight you're placing on your seat. A narrow saddle also allows you to pedal briskly without the annoyance of having your legs bumping into the back and sides of your seat.

Once you've figured out the right saddle width, take some time to get to know the nose (the long narrow body and front) of your saddle. This is where most riders run into trouble in the long term. The nose of your saddle supports your groin and helps you to control and steer the bike. Too much pressure on that part of the saddle can cause pain, numbness, chafing, and general irritation. If your crotch feels uncomfortably smashed in the riding position, look for a saddle with a cutout or groove in the nose. This is designed to eliminate the pressure from those sensitive spots. The right bike seat should feel natural and comfortable right out of the gate (and many, many miles later). If it doesn't, keep looking until you find one that does.

All that said, if you're brand-new to cycling, be forewarned that your butt will be tender in the very beginning. It happens to even seasoned cyclists who take a couple of months off during the winter. Proper cycling shorts (as you'll see in the next section) help tremendously but probably won't take away all the sting. As your glute muscles toughen up, the discomfort will subside. You can make the "break-in" period less painful by easing into riding. Try pedaling 15 to 20 minutes a day until you get used to it. The feeling goes away quickly, and you should be ready to roll in comfort within a week or two.

One final note about butt comfort: Riders of all shapes and sizes sometimes suffer some chafing when the tender skin of their butt rubs against the chamois of their shorts or against the saddle. Larger riders sometimes have more chafing troubles because there's more weight pressing the skin onto the shorts and saddle. You can avoid unwanted sore spots by applying a cream, such as Chamois Butt'r, to the padding in your shorts. It provides a smooth gliding surface and reduces friction so you're less likely to chafe.

✳KITTING UP

Finding cycling clothes for an extra-large frame used to be an exercise in futility. Even if you could find something that fit, you could be pretty sure it wasn't going to be flattering. Though there still isn't an abundance of plus-size riding attire, the pickings are far better than they used to be, as stylish companies like Louis Garneau and Canari have begun offering high-end shorts, jerseys, and tights in Clydesdale and Athena sizes that range up to 3XL. Though it can be a little intimidating to step out of the house in form-fitting Lycra when you're XXL, high-quality, well-tailored cycling clothes not only help you look better on your bike but also, because they're designed specifically for cycling performance, help you ride better. The following are a few essentials that will improve your cycling experience, no matter what your size.

Shorts/bibs. If you splurge on nothing else, invest in the best cycling shorts and/or bibs you can afford. For unsurpassed comfort, especially for larger riders who may have trouble with elastic waistbands digging into their skin or, worse, shorts slipping down while they ride, bib shorts— shorts held up by integrated suspender-style straps—are the way to go. Most bibs come in sizes up to XXL, and companies like Campagnolo make bib shorts up to 3XL. Unfortunately, it's harder for women to find women-specific bibs (which usually have a cross-your-heart-style strap) in extra-large sizes, but men's bibs work just fine. For mountain bike shorts, which often come in baggy, relaxed styles, companies like Hoss offer 3XL.

Jersey. You don't really need a special shirt for cycling, but once you ride in a cycling-specific jersey, you'll never want to pedal in a plain T-shirt again. Cycling jerseys are constructed from special wicking materials that keep you dry and comfortable as you spin down the road. They're also equipped with a zipper in the front for cooling off when the going gets hot and convenient pockets in the back for stashing your cell phone, some cash, a little food, or whatever else you might need for a long ride. They're also tailored to be longer in the back, so you stay covered when you bend forward in the riding position. Many companies offer plus-size jerseys these days.

It's always a good idea to try before you buy, since jerseys come in many different "cuts," from American to European and club to racing. Each is tailored with a slightly different fit, so you'll need to find the one that works for your body type, notes Phyllis. "Even now that I'm down to a size 12–14, race cuts can be difficult for me. American is okay. Club cut can be baggy. I'm a large in European cut and a medium in American. My advice: Try everything before buying."

Arm/knee warmers. If you're new to the sport, these may seem like a superfluous accessory, but any seasoned cyclist will assure you they're a must-have for extending your cycling wardrobe without shelling out a ton of money. As the name implies, arm and knee warmers are sleeves that you pull on under your jersey and shorts to keep your extremities warm during chilly rides. Arm warmers, in particular, are useful because you may start a ride in the morning when it might be 60 degrees, thinking you need long sleeves, but find yourself sweltering in 75-degree temps, wishing for a short-sleeve jersey three-quarters of the way through. With arm warmers you have the best of both worlds. Knee warmers keep your hinges from getting cold when temperatures fall below 65 and save you from buying knicker-length tights. Most companies make arm and knee warmers in XL sizes.

Shoes. New cyclists are always surprised that there are special shoes for cycling; but once you get a taste of the power transfer you get while pedaling in cycling-specific shoes, you'll toss your tennis shoes for good. Cycling shoes have stiff soles that direct all the power you are applying with your legs directly into your pedals, which in turn propels your bike forward with greater ease. The stiff sole also prevents your foot from flexing with every revolution, which helps prevent cramping and foot fatigue on long rides. Cycling shoes are designed to work with clipless pedals, which are special pedal platforms that attach, or click in, to cleats that you screw into the soles of your shoes. The beauty of clipless pedals is that you use the energy from your upstroke (when your leg is coming up and around) as well as that from your downstroke (when your leg is pushing down and back) while you pedal, so every second of saddle time is put to good use. Cycling shoes are often narrow, but more manufacturers are offering wider sizing. One of the best is Sidi, whose shoes come in sizes up to 52, in three widths.

Gloves. You'll see plenty of riders going bare-handed, and gloves more than any accessory are a personal preference. But heavier riders tend to like the extra padding they provide. Remember how your weight is evenly distributed among hands, feet, and rear? If you have extra weight on your upper body, that means stress on your palms, which can lead to tingling and numbness. Additionally, gloves absorb sweat, so you don't slip on your handlebars when it's warm, and they provide extra protection in the event you should take a tumble.

Helmet. If you ride a bike, you need a helmet, period. The good news is it shouldn't be hard to find one that fits, and you won't be forced to pay any extra for it. In fact, top companies like Giro make very reasonably priced helmets that fit hat sizes up to 64 centimeters (cm) for less than 50 bucks.

PICK YOUR COMPONENTS

Most components, which include brakes, shifters, pedals, saddle, and all the other parts on your bike aside from the frame and fork, will suit heavy riders without fail. But if you're in the 230-pound-and-above range, you'll want to pay special attention to a few key components, like handlebars and pedals, which can be made too thin and light for heavier riders.

In general, you want to shy away from titanium, which may sound counterintuitive given the metal's reputation for brute strength. However, manufacturers often make titanium parts extremely thin because they can, says Cushionbury, and that leaves it vulnerable to breaking. Ditto for carbon fiber components. "Sticking to aluminum for bike parts and steel for pedals will work for most riders," he says. "That doesn't mean you have to sacrifice quality. There are plenty of great, strong parts and components that perform well, hold up, and won't really weigh you down." Here's what to look for where it matters most.

Handlebar and stem. The bar is the part you hold on to. The stem is the part that attaches the bar to your bike. Both are obviously very important, and neither will win you that much speed for saving grams with ultralight versions. Instead, go with tried-and-true aluminum (or alloy) bars and stems by manufacturers like Bontrager and Easton.

Pedals. Even light riders can (and do) break flimsy pedals. The part you want to pay close attention to is the pedal spindle, the skinny part that attaches the platform to your crank arm. That should be steel. A reliable brand that exemplifies strong pedals is Shimano.

Saddle. Once you find a comfortable saddle, just be sure it stands up to Clydesdale standards. Almost any metal saddle rails (the parts beneath the saddle that attach to your bike) should be fine, but steer clear of carbon fiber.

Seatpost. This is the tube that your saddle attaches to and can be adjusted up and down to set your seat height. Again, the post itself should be constructed from a strong aluminum (not carbon fiber). Also look for a two-bolt saddle rail clamp system; it's stronger than one bolt, and your saddle will be less likely to shift under your weight.

Wheels. Not to be confused with the tires (the rubber part that rolls on the ground), the wheels are the part of the bike that consists of tire, hub, and spokes. As mentioned earlier, the wheels are the first to fail under extreme weight. So look for 36-spoke construction and go with a strong alloy material, like Mavic alloy-rimmed wheels.

If you're unsure about anything, ask the sales representative at your bike shop to help you pick the right bike and parts for your needs. For a complete guide to cycling gear of all kinds, including where to find the bikes, clothes, tools, and accessories you need, check out the gear section of Bicycling.com at www.bicycling.com/gear.

WHAT ELSE YOU NEED

This program focuses on riding, so your bike is by far the most essential piece of equipment. To accelerate your progress, both in the realm of weight loss and as a rider, you'll also be doing a small amount of cross-training in the form of strength-training. But don't worry. You won't need a pricey gym membership, just a few accessories, two or three pairs of dumbbells (see below), and a large inflated stability ball. The following bike and non-bike-related gear will enhance your training and help you peel off pounds faster.

Bike computer. You don't need more than a plain old watch to start the programs in *Ride Your Way Lean*. But at some point, you'll likely want to invest in a cycling computer. These gadgets work like a sophisticated odometer for your bike. A small screen affixes to your handlebar, and a little sensor attaches to a spoke on your front wheel. From there, you get all kinds of information about your ride, including speed, max speed, average speed, distance, time, and more. Some fancy models include GPS technology, so you can map your ride, and can also tell you the temperature, altitude, and more. Mostly they're fun to have because they're an easy way to track your progress and see how much fitter and faster you're getting. If you start doing charity rides, they're almost essential, so you can follow along on the cue sheets.

Riders who are gunning for weight loss often like to use a cycling computer that works with a heart rate monitor (see page 58), which, along with all the other statistics on your ride, will tell you how many calories you've burned. Keeping track of the energy you use on each ride is a great way to manage the calories you take in and may help you lose weight faster.

Weights. To perform the strength-training moves, you'll need at least two sets of dumbbells: one set for upper-body moves and a heavier set for lower-body moves. How much weight you'll need varies widely from person to person. Generally, women will use weights in the 8- to 20-pound range, and men will use weights in the 15- to 30-pound range.

You can save yourself floor space (and the hassle of buying more weights) by investing in adjustable-weight dumbbell sets like Reebok Speed Pac. These all-in-one weights contain small weight plates that attach to a handle. To adjust the weight you're going to lift, you simply move a pin that attaches more or fewer of the weight plates, while the rest stay nestled in the platform holder.

Stability ball. Many of these moves also require a stability ball. You can find these large inflatable balls (which also go under the name Swiss ball) at most department and sporting good stores. Stability balls are excellent training tools for cyclists because they also challenge and improve your sense of balance, which, of course, directly benefits how you handle yourself on a bike. Read the sizing chart on the label to find the right ball size for your height. When you sit on the ball, your hips should be level or just slightly higher than your knees. Balls typically come in sizes 55 cm for people (4'11"–5'4"), 65 cm (5'5"–5'11"), and 75 cm (6'0"–6'7").

If you're very overweight, you may be concerned about the ball holding your weight. Many companies, like Ball Dynamics and SPRI, offer balls that can hold 600-plus pounds. Just read the packaging before purchasing if you're concerned.

Scale. Nothing says commitment to weight loss like a scale. Part of the success of programs like Weight Watchers are the weekly weigh-ins that force you to be accountable. But anyone who's ever lost weight knows the scale can be both motivating and discouraging.

"When I was heavy, getting on the scale was torture," recalls Phyllis. "I got to a certain point where I just skipped getting on the damn thing—just too depressing—and I didn't care how fat I was." Eventually she realized she had to know the numbers if she really wanted to take the weight off. "I would get on every couple of weeks to see if my progress was heading in the right direction," she recalls. "Then I joined Weight Watchers, and the only time I would get on was at the meetings." Today she uses the scale for maintenance. "I mostly rely on the 'belt-o-meter,'" she says. "If I feel like my pants are getting tight, I get on the scale to see how tight they are. If I've picked up 3 pounds or more, I start journaling what I eat and paying attention to [Weight Watchers] points until those pounds go bye-bye. The scale is still not my friend, but I don't dread getting on it. It's just part of my training."

You can buy an everyday bathroom scale from your local department store. Or go with a fancy body composition one, like the models offered by Tanita. If you go the body composition route, remember that those scales are very sensitive to hydration status and have a fairly modest margin of error, so don't get extremely hung up on those numbers; use them as a general guide.

Food and exercise logs. A simple journal can prove to be your most potent exercise tool. A recent study of more than 1,600 overweight adults found that those who kept logs of their food intake and exercise habits lost twice as much weight over a 6-month period as those who didn't keep written track.

You can download free diet and exercise logs online, buy inexpensive paper versions at your local bookstore, or enroll in an online service that allows you to record your workouts and food intake on a daily spreadsheet. No matter which method you choose, you're bound to get better results than if you skip this important, powerful step.

3:GET FIT FASTER

HOW TO USE YOUR BIKE AS THE ULTIMATE WEIGHT-LOSS TOOL

ABOUT 5 YEARS ago, I took a new client out riding. She was about 60 pounds overweight and had been on every diet and exercise plan known to man. Inspired by my complete love for cycling, she had bought a bike and had been riding pretty regularly for about 3 months. I wanted to take her through a few workouts to help ramp up her results. "Okay, we're going to pedal as fast as we can for 30 seconds," I began instructing. She looked at me and said, dead seriously, "I don't think I want to do speedwork. I don't care about getting faster. I just want to burn fat."

I can't tell you how many times I've seen riders back off from going hard to stay in the fat-burning zone. Don't get me wrong. There's a time, a place, and a purpose for low-intensity rides. And yes, that type of riding does dip primarily into your fat stores. But steadfastly riding at slower speeds won't whittle your waist the way you may have been told. The best use of two wheels to lose weight includes a variety of rides and riding intensities, from beach cruiser slow to blazingly fast.

Just ask Jason Blessing, 38, of Lake Tahoe, California, a software company executive with 6-year-old triplets. He lost 55 pounds, dropping from 260 to 205, in 7 months by learning how to make the most of his limited riding time. "I've been riding on and off since my mid-teens. But after I got further into my professional life, I had less time to ride, and the weight started piling on," he recalls. Then he met coach James Herrera (who helped craft the weight-loss plans in this book), who turned him on to interval training. "Now I get up early and do an hour spin in the morning before work, and I make the most of that hour by doing intervals. It's helped tremendously with the weight loss, and it also improved my fitness a lot. Before I even lost all the weight, I was so much faster when I did my weekend rides. I was a good 15 minutes faster up Tunnel Creek [a local 3-mile mountain bike climb] this year. I didn't have to stop and catch my breath like before. There are always ways to fit in a workout and to make it count."

Here's a look at how cycling burns fat and calories and how to make your bike your best weight-loss tool.

FIRST, LET'S BURN SOME CALORIES

Riding a bike burns calories—hundreds and thousands of them—even when you don't feel like you're working terribly hard. The chart (opposite), from "The Compendium of Physical Activities Tracking Guide," which was developed by a doctor from Stanford University to standardize these measurements, shows how many calories a 150-pound rider burns every hour for various kinds of riding. If you want to figure out how many calories you'll burn, take your weight and divide it by 2.2 to express it in kilograms. Then multiply that number by the METS (metabolic equivalents, a unit of the energy cost of an activity) number in parentheses. That's how many calories you'll burn in an hour.

RIDING AT . . .	BURNS . . .
Less than 10 mph, very leisurely	272 calories (4 METS)
10–12 mph, easy	408 calories (6 METS)
12–14 mph, moderate	544 calories (8 METS)
14–16 mph, vigorous	680 calories (10 METS)
16–19 mph, very fast	816 calories (12 METS)
More than 20 mph, racing speed	1,088 calories (16 METS)

You can see how your calorie burn grows exponentially with your effort. That's because the faster you go, the harder it is to go even faster. Air drag, which is what you have to overcome as you pedal down the road, is proportional to the square of speed—which is a very scientific way to say that you have to work dramatically harder to go fast as your speed increases because you have to overcome higher wind resistance. That's why riders wear all that funny gear, like the long pointed helmet and shoe covers, when they race in time trials. They're trying to cheat the wind in every way possible.

From the chart you also can see the benefits of performing intervals. Even if you can ride really fast only for short bursts, you can still dramatically increase your calorie burn. Additionally, intervals increase your lactate threshold (the point at which your legs start to burn and you slow down), so you become a faster rider overall, which, of course, means a bigger total calorie burn.

Finally, cycling also helps you burn more calories long after you've racked your bike. Exercise researchers have found that your metabolism stays higher for up to 12 hours after a vigorous workout, which adds up to about 15 bonus calories for every 100 calories that you burned during exercise. Some riders take advantage of this afterburn phenomenon by doing two rides on days when there's time, performing a short spin in the morning and another later in the day.

✳WHERE THOSE CALORIES COME FROM

Now let's address the whole "ride slow to burn more fat" philosophy. Whenever you ride (or do any exercise), your body uses both fat and carbohydrate for fuel. (Protein is generally used to maintain and repair your muscle tissue and isn't usually used for fuel.) How much of either it uses is a sliding scale that depends on how hard and long you ride.

Fat, as you might expect, is your body's endurance fuel. When you're spinning along at a very mellow pace (about 50 percent of your max heart rate; see page 60), your body has enough stored fat to fuel activity for hours, maybe even days. The problem is it takes longer to pull fat out of storage and burn it for fuel. So as you pick up the pace, your body needs faster fuel, which means carbohydrates. Stored carbohydrate (glycogen) is your body's preferred fuel for moderate- to high-intensity rides. You're still burning some fat, but considerably less as exercise intensity ramps up. Glycogen is a very effective energy source, but unlike fat, you don't have a bottomless supply. Most of us have enough glycogen stocked away in our muscles to fuel about 2 hours of spirited riding. After that, the well runs dry, and you get that vapory feeling (called the "bonk" in cycling circles), and either have to eat something quickly or resort to dramatically reducing your intensity to go back to fat-burning mode.

Reading all that, you may assume, as many of my clients (and a surprising number of trainers) do, that slow-speed riding is best for burning off unwanted fat. What they're missing in this equation is the calorie factor. If you want to lose weight, your main goal should be burning calories, which is what high-intensity exercise does best. Consider this: If you ride for an hour at an easy pace, you'll burn about 450 calories, 270 of them from fat. Now, let's say you ride vigorously for that same hour. You'll burn 640 calories, about 250 of them from fat. In the end you've burned nearly 200 more calories and almost equal amounts of fat.

You can accomplish your weight-loss goals either way. You can ride more leisurely, but just ride longer, which is easier when you ride leisurely, to burn more calories. Or you can ride harder for less time to accomplish the same result. Since most people don't always have the time to go long or the energy and fitness to go really hard all the time, the best strategy incorporates both. Just remember that when it comes to shedding pounds, it's energy expenditure—no matter where that energy comes from—that counts most.

✳GROW YOUR FAT-BURNING ENGINES

While it's true that you don't have to burn stored fat for fuel to shed fat from your body, one of the beauties of cycling, as mentioned in Chapter 1, is it will make you a better fat-burning machine. As you ride more and improve your fitness, your body becomes more adept at burning fat even at higher riding intensities.

There's even a scientific name for this transformation. It's called the crossover concept. It's when your body switches over and starts using more fat and fewer carbohydrates for fuel during endurance exercise. This crossover happens because of a cascade of training adaptations. For one, your body creates more fatty-acid-binding proteins, which help shuttle fatty acids from storage into your working muscles. To better burn those fatty acids, your body pumps out higher levels of carnitine transferase, an enzyme that helps those fatty acids cross the membrane of your cell's power generators, which are known as mitochondria. To speed the delivery and accommodate the load of all these free fatty acids, your body "builds more roads," by extending more capillaries within your muscles. Finally, it makes your fat-burning mitochondria bigger and stronger to help you burn the increased load of fatty acids flowing into your muscles.

One of the big benefits of being a better fat burner is you can ride much longer on less fuel, which means you're burning stored fat and hundreds of calories without feeling ravenous. That's the secret behind lean pro cyclists, explains Allen Lim, PhD, a physiologist who has trained many successful pro cyclists and works with Lance Armstrong at Team Radio Shack. Through training and dietary changes (which you'll learn more about in Chapter 5), he found that even his most bonk-prone riders could go for 6 hours in the saddle with unopened energy bars in their jersey pockets.

The plans in this book are specially formulated to maximize this cross-over process. They include just the right blend of hard, short workouts that raise your fitness ceiling, so your easy cruising speed becomes steadily faster, with longer, more moderate workouts that stimulate the growth of a spider-web of capillaries and beef up your mitochondria, all of which improve your fat-burning ability. The end result is you get faster and fitter in less time.

No matter where you're starting, it's never, ever too late to learn or to reap enormous benefits. At age 58, Carol Goodman of Boulder, Colorado, recalls weighing a "grim 303 pounds" and one day just deciding that she'd had enough. She wanted to start exercising and finally get healthy, but her knees wouldn't let her walk very fast or far, let alone try a typical cardio class. Her husband suggested a bike. "It was a virtual miracle on two wheels," she recalls. She spent 16 months building up her endurance, strength, and stamina. Four years later, she weighs 163 pounds and does long rides whenever she can. "My only regret is waiting so long to experience the joy of cycling."

CRANK OUT THE RIGHT CADENCE

To maximize your cycling comfort and efficiency, it helps to ride with the right cadence. Cadence is your pedaling speed as measured in revolutions per minute (rpm), how many times you turn the pedals around in a full circle each minute. Before Lance Armstrong made his postcancer comeback, often spinning his pedals at a dizzying 110 rpm, mainstream cyclists didn't pay a tremendous amount of attention to their pedaling cadence. Post Lance, high-speed cadence became all the rage. These days, the school of thought seems to be settling into the middle ground, with the "best" cadence depending on your physiology and cycling goals.

Each time you push on your pedals, your muscular system kicks in to produce power, and your cardiovascular system fires up to deliver oxygen and fuel to your muscles and to clear metabolic waste, like lactic acid, that you produce as you ride. The cadence you select should allow you to balance both of these systems without either one burning out before the ride is done.

Novice riders generally make the mistake of mashing a big gear at low rpm because they feel as if they should be working hard every minute they ride. I've actually had many a client complain that pedaling in the gear I suggested felt too easy; however, after 30 minutes, they appreciated the advice. When you ride in a hard gear, you're making your muscles work hard, as they would when you're strength-training, which, as you might imagine, causes your legs to fatigue pretty fast. To get the idea, think about how you work your muscles in a weight room. You can likely lift a 35-pound dumbbell, but probably not too many times before your muscles cry uncle and need a rest because they're producing more metabolic waste than they can clear. Pick up a 10-pound dumbbell, however, and you can lift and lower it many times over before you tire out. The same applies to the work your muscles are doing on your bike. By pedaling at a lower gear at a higher cadence, you're spreading out the workload and making it easier for your legs to pedal over and over, so you can ride longer and burn more fat and calories than you would if you were forcing your muscles to work very hard for each pedal stroke.

New research shows that slow, hard pedaling also empties out your glycogen stores at a faster rate than brisk, more moderate spinning. In a University of Wisconsin and University of Wyoming study of trained cyclists, researchers had riders pedal at 50 rpm in a hard gear for 30 minutes, then repeated the test another day—only this time they had the cyclists pedal an easier gear at 100 rpm. Though their power output and oxygen consumption were about the same in both tests, they burned through their precious glycogen stores much more quickly when mashing a monster gear, and they burned far more fat for fuel when quickly pedaling an easier gear. Since you have limited amounts of glycogen to spare, that's another reason slow, hard pedaling is just too difficult to sustain.

That said, faster is not always better. Spinning way too fast can actually slow you down and burn you out as quickly as gear mashing. A Spanish study of well-trained cyclists that compared the efficiency and power output of riders pedaling 80, 100, and 120 rpm found that when the cyclists hit 120 rpm, their watts (the amount of power they produced) dropped by 9 percent while their breathing rate increased (read: they were gasping for air). For many riders, a super-high cadence is also less effective because their brain can't coordinate their movements quickly enough to maintain control and their legs end up flailing while they bounce around in the saddle. Nothing efficient about that.

What's the sweet spot? For most riders it's somewhere in the 80 to 100 rpm range, the place where you can pedal fast, but in control, while still applying a moderate, sustainable amount of pressure on the pedals. (Obviously, your cadence will drop when going uphill, which is fine.) There are some bike computers that will tell you your cadence, but you can also simply count. To count your cadence, use a stopwatch to count the number of times your leg pushes down on the pedal for 30 seconds and multiply by 2. Or if that is too difficult to do while you ride, just count for 10 seconds and multiply by 6. Once you get the hang of what various cadences feel like, it will become automatic to use your shifting to keep your cadence in a quick and comfortable range.

If your cadence is low, say below 80, try to increase it. How high depends on your physiology. The riders who benefit from a higher-end cadence are generally lighter riders, women, master (older) cyclists, and others whose aerobic capacity tends to be greater than their muscle power. As a general rule when you're starting out, if your legs are giving out before your lungs, increase your cadence. If you're gasping for breath but your legs are fine, lower it. Practice will help you improve your cadence and find the right rpm for you. Here are a few other tips.

Shift often. Unless you live where it's pancake flat, you'll want to use your gears to help keep your cadence comfortable. If you're new to cycling, it can take a little time and practice before your shifting becomes automatic. In the meantime, try to feel and anticipate the ride. As you feel the pressure on your pedals increasing, whether it's a small rise or a stiff headwind, shift down to an easier gear. When you feel your legs starting to "spin out" because of a slight downhill or tailwind, shift up into a harder gear. The more you can anticipate your shifting needs (especially on climbs), the smoother and steadier your riding (and cadence) will be.

Pedal circles. The term *spinning* comes from the motion your legs should make while you pedal. Whether you use toe clips or clipless pedals, you want to concentrate on pulling up on your pedals as they're coming around as much as you push down on them. It should feel like a smooth, fluid rotation.

Be patient. Remember, quick-cadence pedaling is a very aerobic activity. So if you're fresh off the couch without a lot of cardiovascular conditioning, you may find yourself feeling out of breath more quickly than you'd like. Ease into it by gradually picking up your pedal speed, and your legs will become faster as you become fitter.

Make some muscle. Cycling-specific strength-training (see Chapter 7) has been shown to improve your riding efficiency at nearly every cadence because it increases your strength, so you can generate more power per pedal stroke.

Coast less. Keep those pedals turning whenever possible. Sure, there'll be some steep descents and some stopping and starting, where coasting is necessary on any ride. But make a concerted effort to use your gears to keep power going into your pedals on 90 percent of your ride. This is good advice for burning more calories as well as improving cadence.

✳BUILD YOUR CYCLING STRENGTH

Again, cycling is a power-to-weight sport. We're already working on the backside of that equation. But it's not all about weight. Take a gander at some of the sprinters in a bike race or check out a group of track cyclists, and you'll quickly see that you don't need to be skinny to go really, really fast. You also can make considerable progress and have more fun riding by working on building your power. Resistance training is one way, and we'll give complete details in Chapter 7, but there are many ways to build power while on the bike. Though you can create muscle mass more effectively in the gym, on-the-bike strength training has the advantage of making this muscle mass more functional for riding. In other words, the muscle you make is very, very specific to the goal you want to accomplish—getting faster.

Some experts have set the optimal power-to-weight standard (for recreational athletes) as the ability to produce 1.6 watts of power per pound of body weight. So if you weigh 180 pounds, you should be able to crank out 288 watts for over 45 minutes. Here are a few ways to pump more power into your pedals.

Note: Since these drills put a higher load on your joints, especially your knees, you should have a month of resistance training under your belt before incorporating them.

Resistance intervals. No sooner do we tell you to speed it up, than we're going to tell you to slow it down. But as mentioned earlier, building muscle strength, torque, and power will help you pedal more effectively at every cadence. Resistance intervals do just that. The upside is many heavier riders love these drills because they play to their strengths. These workouts are best done inside with your bike mounted on an indoor trainer (see Chapter 6), or outside on a steady, slight incline.

After a good warmup (10 minutes at an easy to moderate pace), click into a harder gear or start your incline until you are pedaling against a resistance that slows your cadence to 55 to 65 rpm. Your heart rate will be lower, while your muscle contraction will be much higher. Concentrate on keeping your pedal stroke smooth and circular. Ride this way for 5 to 6 minutes. Recover for $2^{1}/_{2}$ to 3 minutes (half the interval time). Repeat 2 to 3 times. Gradually work your way up to 10-minute intervals done 4 or 5 times with 5 minutes of recovery in between. These fall under Zones 3 and 4 in Chapter 4.

Jump starts. These drills mimic a standing sprint start. They help to increase your power to your pedals and are fun to do. After a good warmup, find a long stretch of flat road (you can also do these on an indoor trainer), and shift into a high gear that is very hard to turn over, so you are pedaling very, very slowly (about 5 mph). Give yourself a countdown and then jump out of the saddle and start driving the pedals down as hard as possible. Continue for 10 to 12 seconds. Shift back into a lighter gear and spin easy for about 5 minutes to recover. Repeat for a set of 3 to 5 jumps, gradually building up to 8 to 10 jumps. These fall under Zones 4 and 5 in Chapter 4.

Kick-it-up sprints. After a good warmup, shift into a high gear that you can still spin relatively easily. Begin sprinting; after 5 to 10 seconds shift into a harder gear, then repeat after another 5 to 10 seconds, and then one more time, finishing the sprint out in a challenging gear for a total of a 30-second sprint. Spin easy in a lighter gear for about 10 minutes. Then repeat two more times. These fall under Zones 4 and 5 in Chapter 4.

Seated climbing. Nothing will make you stronger faster than climbing. These seated climbing drills are similar to resistance intervals, except they're longer and done at a higher, more variable cadence. Ideally, these are done on a long, gradual (4 to 6 percent grade) climb that takes 20 to 30 minutes to crest. But if you don't have that kind of sustained hill in your neck of the woods, you can always do hill repeats—go up, come back down, repeating until you've achieved 20 to 30 minutes of climbing time.

After a good warmup, approach the climb and, staying seated, begin to climb in a moderate gear at about 80 rpm. After 5 minutes, shift into a harder gear and slow your cadence to about 65 rpm. Five minutes later, shift to an easier gear and pick up your cadence. Continue alternating all the way to the top of the climb. By alternating, you improve your power and endurance across the spectrum of resistance and cadence. These fall under Zones 3 and 4 in Chapter 4.

✳CLIMB LIKE A CHAMPION

Hills. They are at once a cyclist's nemesis and ally. We hate them. We love them. We love to hate them. And no matter which side of the fence we fall on during a given ascent, they always make us stronger. And they burn megacalories. Climbing scorches 8 to 10 calories a minute for a 150-pound rider (much more than that for heavier cyclists). Though grappling against the force of gravity is undoubtedly more difficult when you have extra weight that isn't helping to push the pedals, climbing isn't easy for any rider, big or small. Everyone just suffers at a different rate. That said, there are techniques you can use to make even the longest, steepest climbs just a little bit easier.

Gear down for it. Anticipate the climb by shifting into an easier gear from the get-go. New riders often try to muscle up a climb, then quickly learn that it's pretty difficult to recover on a hill once your legs are loaded up with metabolic waste. Try to keep your cadence between 70 and 80 rpm. The goal is to balance the work of your legs with that of your lungs. They should both be putting out pretty equal efforts. When you find the right cadence, you should feel like you are working but not being throttled.

Assume the power position. The key to comfortable climbing is maximizing your muscle power and your oxygen flow. That means staying seated. Though you do generate more power when you stand because your full body weight is pushing down on the pedals, your heart rate is higher, and it takes about 10 percent more energy overall, because your upper body has to work to support your torso and your legs need to support your full body weight. Heavier riders have to use even more energy because there's more weight to support. That's why you generally see only very light cyclists spending a lot of time climbing out of the saddle.

Though you normally want to ride in the lowest position comfortably possible to minimize wind resistance, the opposite is true when you climb. You want to sit as tall as possible to encourage maximum airflow into your lungs. Position your hands on the top of your handlebar, so they're about shoulder width apart. Drop your elbows and relax your upper body, keeping your shoulders back and chest open. Try to keep your upper body still and relaxed, as you pull back on the bars and press through your pedals. Any tension or side-to-side movement just wastes energy. To gain more leverage from each pedal stroke, shift your weight back on your saddle, so you get more pushing power from your large glute and hip muscles. Remember to keep your cadence high, spinning rather than mashing up the incline.

Take a stand. All that said, there are times when it makes sense to get out of the saddle for a stretch. On long, steep climbs standing occasionally will give your body a much-needed break because it uses different muscle groups. Standing can also help you power over short, steep pitches more quickly than if you remain seated. It also just feels good to stretch out your legs.

For the best results, place your hands on the brake hoods for leverage. Shift into the next hardest gear just before you stand, to take advantage of the extra power you generate when you stand and to maintain a steady pace during the transition. Pull on the bars and allow the bike to rock side to side underneath you. Your body will naturally come forward a little, but try not to lean too far forward, as that just puts more weight on your arms and may cause your rear tire to slip. Keep your weight back, directly over your cranks, so you feel the saddle brushing the back of your legs.

If you're riding with others, be careful to prevent your bike from "kicking back" as you come out of the saddle, because it's pretty easy to hit the rider behind you. This happens because the bike can decelerate briefly as you go from sitting to standing. To counteract this deceleration, just press forward on your bar so your bike doesn't lose momentum. Likewise, when you're ready to sit back down, push the bike forward so it settles beneath you and click into an easier gear to keep your pace smooth and consistent.

Stay in your comfort zone. Ride with other cyclists enough and you'll find that everyone tries to be a hero on the hills. Though it can be fun to go for king of the mountain (KOM) points when you're out with a group, listen to your body and stay within your limits. If you push yourself into the red trying to stay with the better climbers early on the hill, then blow up and need to slow way down, you'll lose much more time overall than if you had just ridden at your own pace to the top. Keep your breathing deep and rhythmic. If you find yourself gasping, you're pushing too hard. And remember, gravity may not be your best friend as you're working your way up the hill, but it sure does you a few favors on the other side. It's very common for light riders to crest a climb first, only to get passed by their heavier counterparts on the downhill.

✳COMMUTE TO KEEP IT COMING

Your bike is fun to ride and a terrific exercise tool, but don't forget that it's also a really great form of transportation. Nothing against cars; they're a necessary part of life in this country. But it's important to note that the massive upswing in obesity rates coincides remarkably with the number of miles we drive today. We now drive an average of 30 miles a day and weigh roughly 30 pounds more than we did in 1960. Sitting in a car, as you might imagine, burns very little energy—about 1 calorie per minute. Riding a bike, even at a very leisurely tooling-around-town pace burns four to six times that amount. You likely have a few places you frequent that are well within bikable distance. Try riding to the store, the library, even work, if the roads are accessible. All those little calories add up. Plus small bursts of exercise during the day keep your metabolism high, and that's good for you.

QUICK CALORIE-BURNING TRICK

Here's a little trick that pro cyclists swear by when they want to fry fat fast: When possible, sneak in an easy 20-minute spin before breakfast. Seasoned cyclists will even set up their trainer in a convenient spot so they can hop on without leaving the comfort of their home. This simple routine not only burns an additional 1,000 calories a week but also turbo-charges your fat-burning metabolism, says Andy Pruitt, EdD, director of the Boulder Center for Sports Medicine in Colorado. "Getting in motion first thing draws on your fat-burning stores and ignites the fat-burning process," he says. "When I was traveling with USA Cycling, the athletes couldn't have breakfast until they'd pedaled 20 minutes." Including this brief second exercise bout in your day boosts levels of circulating growth hormone, which helps build muscle and burn fat.

In a landmark study of more than 67,000 women who were followed for 7 years, researchers found that those who cycled for transportation had lower rates of heart disease, stroke, and cancer, compared with their inactive peers. Similarly, a study of nearly 7,000 men and women found that those who spent an average of 3 hours per week biking to work had a 28 percent lower risk of dying prematurely from any illness than their sedentary counterparts, even if they didn't do any other exercise.

By using your bike to run errands, you're also more likely to shift into active thinking throughout the day. Once you realize you can ride somewhere nearly as quickly as drive (and parking is always much easier), you'll soon see that you can walk places you used to go by car, and you'll start to prefer taking the active route to the sedentary one. As you lose weight, you'll also have more energy and motivation to keep your body moving, as Eric DeLorme, 40, of Orléans, Canada, has recently discovered.

"For years and years I rode lots," recalls Eric. Then he got a "real job," got married, had two kids, and watched his waistline expand from a 35 to a 42 and beyond. "I never weighed myself. Every time I looked in the mirror, I fooled myself into thinking I looked good." Then he went to his doctor for a routine appointment. "What a wake-up! My doc might as well have punched me in the gut: 280 pounds, blood pressure 190/130, and generally ugly blood work. The next day I started commuting by bike. It's about a 50-kilometer round-trip. At first, the 25-kilometer morning ride would take me over 75 minutes. By the end of the summer, I was angry at myself if it took more than 55 minutes (stop time at traffic lights included)."

A few months later and 40 pounds lighter, Eric has shed 5 inches from his waistline and has improved his blood pressure enough to avoid medication. "I'm more pragmatic than dogmatic about commuting. If it rains in the morning, I take the bus. I average about 3 to 4 days a week of commuting most of the year. When the days are short, I ride my trainer to keep the weight off. Cycle commuting will be a permanent part of my long-term weight-maintenance strategy. It has to! Because I'm not buying more fat pants, that's for sure."

4:RIDE IT OFF

ALL THE PLANS YOU NEED FOR ALL THE WEIGHT YOU WANT TO LOSE

TECHNICALLY, YOU DON'T need a plan to ride your way lean. You can just saddle up and ride lots. So long as you're practicing smart eating habits as well, the pounds will likely come off. But I can almost guarantee you that they won't come off quite as quickly as they will when you add a little structure.

A well-crafted plan ensures that you put in quality, not just quantity, time on your bike, maximizing short days, intelligently extending endurance rides, and leaving ample room for rest and recovery. It makes sure you get fit, not fatigued, and that pounds melt off at a steady, sustainable pace rather than all at once as you rocket out of the gate only to creep on again when you eventually burn out. A plan takes the guesswork out of what you should do from day to day, leaving you with more energy to simply unrack your bike and ride.

A structured program is also motivating. You're less likely to blow off riding if you have a specific workout on your calendar. It also gives you a chance to look back and see how much progress you've made as well as look

DO YOU NEED TO SEE A DOC?

Most healthy people don't need to see a doctor before they start training. That's especially true if you've been exercising, even just walking, for a while already. But it's important to take the necessary precautions and see a physician first if you have health problems. If you have been completely sedentary for years, have an existing heart condition, chest pain, dizzy spells, or other potentially dangerous symptoms, get your doc's stamp of approval before you embark on a training program.

forward to what's in store. Once you have a sense of what a structured plan looks and feels like, it's also easier to have the confidence that you know what to do to meet your weight-loss, maintenance, and cycling goals.

This chapter contains four plans: Big Weight Loss (35 to 50+ pounds), Drop a Size or More (15 to 35 pounds), Shed the Stubborn Spare Tire (5 to 15 pounds), and Fit for Life (weight maintenance). Each plan is carefully crafted to deliver the proper blend of mileage, intensity, and endurance to burn through the fat and leave plenty of lean muscle and cardiovascular fitness behind.

THE MAGIC OF TRAINING

All riding is technically "training" since every time you turn your pedals you're burning calories and altering your metabolism. Your body adapts to the exercise challenge by building muscle and becoming more fit. The difference between just riding around and structured training is that structured training is designed to create very specific fitness adaptations that will help you progress toward your goal more effectively.

As mentioned earlier in the discussion of fat burning, the biggest adaptation your body makes in the sport of cycling is its efficiency at using oxygen. The first few times you go out for a ride, your legs will probably burn, and you'll find yourself huffing and puffing up every hill. That's a sign that your body isn't yet very effective at delivering oxygen to your working muscles. In just a few weeks, you'll find that you barely register little hills that once hurt. You'll be able to ride faster and farther without needing to slow or stop to catch your breath. That's when you know that your fitness (and fat burning) is well under way. Here's a snapshot of what's happening inside.

Your heart squeezes harder. Your heart is a fist-shaped muscle that squeezes to pump oxygen-rich blood through your body. As you ride, you challenge your heart to deliver as much blood as it can to your working muscles. Over time it adapts by getting stronger, so it can squeeze out more blood with every beat. This means your heart doesn't have to beat as fast or work as hard as you climb steep hills or chase your friends down the road. You'll notice this off the bike as well. It's common for sedentary men and women to have resting heart rates (typically measured first thing in the morning) of 70 to 80 beats per minute (bpm). As you get more fit, you can expect that number to drop 10 to 15 beats, into the 50 to 60 bpm range, which as you might expect, is better for your general health.

Your network expands. A few years ago, I went to see Body Worlds, the show where they have cadavers engaged in sports and activities to show the truly miraculous work of the human body. There was a cyclist whose legs had been stripped of everything but the capillaries, which were shot with bright red ink. It looked like a thousand Day-Glo spiders had taken up residence in his quads. As you ride more, your legs need all the oxygen-rich blood they can get to help your cells' aerobic energy-making furnaces produce energy. So your body forges thousands of new capillaries into your muscles to maximize your circulation. As the transportation system expands, your body produces more aerobic enzymes that extract oxygen from your blood to help your cells burn fat and make energy.

You raise your ceiling. The end result of these adaptations is that you can stay in an aerobic training zone longer, even when you push the pedals faster and harder. That means you raise your lactate threshold, the point at which your muscles can no longer use oxygen for energy and start blasting away at stored carbs without oxygen (something they can't do for very long before your legs begin to burn too much and you have to slow down). The more you raise your lactate threshold, the faster and harder you can ride before your muscles scream uncle and throw on the brakes, which, of course, means an even greater calorie (and fat) burn at the end of the day.

☀MEASURING YOUR EFFORTS

At the heart of training is knowing how hard—or how easy—you're going. Many cyclists spend too much time in a virtual no-man's-land, where they're going a little harder than they should to build endurance but not hard enough to make meaningful gains in lactate threshold. The result is they sort of get stuck at one speed. Even if you don't care how fast you're going or never intend to race, measuring your efforts and building your fitness will help you lose weight and get fit faster.

There are a number of ways to measure intensity. For this program we'll focus on two: heart rate and breathing, the latter being the only one you really need.

☀THE "BREATH-ALYZER"

Want to know how hard you're going? Pay attention to your breathing. Since your muscles need more or less oxygen depending on how hard you're riding, the way you're breathing is a direct indication of how much work you're doing. James Herrera, who developed the weight-loss plans in this chapter, swears by this method for athletes of all levels. "Nothing gives you an instant and honest evaluation of your effort like your breathing," he says.

To make this method even more accurate, pair it with rate of perceived exertion (RPE), a technical way of saying: On a scale of 1 to 10, how hard are you working? A 1 is coasting along a wide-open road with the wind at your back, barely pushing the pedals. A 10 is racing up a steep mountainside as though fleeing wild dogs. You rate how hard you're riding by ranking your effort on a scale between the two extremes. Scientists devised RPE as a way to measure exercise intensity, and studies show it works just as well as heart rate monitoring and other equipment when you use it properly. The key is that you have to pay attention so you don't inadvertently allow yourself to push too hard or slack off for too long. That's why it works best in conjunction with monitoring your breathing. You don't stop breathing, so it's always there as a reminder to check your efforts.

Herrera recommends following this scale:

Zone 1: Light and relaxed breathing—barely above normal. It's an RPE of 1 to 2.

Zone 2: Deep, steady, relaxed breathing. That's your aerobic, endurance-training zone. It's an RPE of 3 to 4.

Zone 3: Slightly labored. This is a steady "tempo" pace, where you're working just a hair above your endurance comfort zone. It's where you'd be if you were riding with someone just slightly faster than you. It's an RPE of 5 to 6.

Zone 4: Short, quick, rhythmic breathing. This is your lactate threshold zone, right where you're hitting your sustainable upper limits. Also known as race pace, it's an RPE of 7 to 8.

Zone 5: Hard, gasping-for-breath breathing. This is your VO$_2$ max training zone, which is a fancy way of saying the top of your limit, as hard as you can go. It's an RPE of 9 to 10.

FOLLOW YOUR HEART

Heart rate monitoring is like reading the electric meter on your house. The higher the number you rack up, the more energy you're using while you're spinning down the road. Heart rate monitoring was once the gold standard for measuring exercise intensity. Pro racers now use power meters (which measure power output in watts) as well, but heart rate remains a popular and potent and affordable training tool.

To measure heart rate, you need a heart rate monitor. If you've never used one, it's a two-part device. The first part is a transmitter that sits on your breastbone right over your heart and is fixed there with a strap that wraps around your torso. The second part is a computer readout that acts as a cardiovascular dashboard. You mount this computer to your handlebar (you can also wear it as a watch), and the sensor on your chest picks up the signal from your heart and transmits it to the computer so you can see how many beats your heart is thumping per minute. Most models also let you program your training zones and will beep if you fall below or push past your target zone.

If you invest in a heart rate monitor, you'll find instructions for setting your training zones based off your maximum heart rate (MHR), the highest number of beats your heart can pump out in 1 minute. Many will offer two options for calculating your max. One is the old "220 minus your age formula" (so if you're 40, your MHR is 180). The other is to strap on the sensor and take an exercise test that will actually tell you your max heart rate. The age formula is okay, but as you would expect, there's a pretty fair margin of error. If you can, take the test. Once you've determined your max, break your heart rate down into training zones to accomplish goals including endurance training, lactate threshold training, and recovery. Calculate your zones based on your MHR. For instance, a recovery heart rate for the 40-year-old rider mentioned above would be less than 115 bpm (180 [MHR] × 0.64 [% of MHR] = 115). This chart shows how heart rate zones coincide with the breathing/RPE zones described above.

TRAINING ZONE	% MHR	RPE
Zone 1 (recovery, easy day)	60–64	1–2
Zone 2 (aerobic endurance)	65–74	3–4
Zone 3 (high-level aerobic, "tempo pace")	75–84	5–6
Zone 4 (lactate threshold, race pace)	85–94	7–8
Zone 5 (max effort)	95–100	9–10

Because of the exact numbers and percentages, heart rate monitoring looks like an exact science. But don't be fooled. Different coaches use different heart rate formulas and training zones. There's also a great deal of variation from one rider to the next. You may hit your lactate threshold (LT) at 75 percent, while more seasoned cyclists don't bump their LT ceiling until they reach 85 percent.

No matter how faithful you are as a person, your heart is also bound to be a little fickle. Your bpm can drift up or down depending on how many times you stopped at Starbucks today (caffeine, as you may have guessed, raises heart rate), whether it's cold or hot outside, and how late you stayed up the night before. Given its capricious nature, it's not always the perfect indicator of performance. For the best results, always pair heart rate with your breathing and RPE. It'll give you a more complete picture of what's going on.

TRAINING EFFORTS

Now that you have all the tools you need to monitor your efforts, you need some efforts to actually monitor. The hallmark of training is working your body at varying intensities to accomplish specific fitness, and in this case, weight-loss, goals. That means intervals—and lots of 'em. By pushing your body outside of your comfort zone over and over, you get fitter faster and burn more calories as your body becomes accustomed to working at higher intensities.

For example, let's say that when you start out you can ride 15 miles on your local recreation path in just over an hour, averaging 14 to 15 miles per hour (mph). By incorporating intervals, where you ride several-minute bouts at 16 to 17 mph (with periods of recovery between), you'll make your body gradually adapt to the harder effort, so soon you will be able to sustain it for the entire ride. You've effectively raised your cruising speed. Here are the types of intervals you'll be doing in the *Ride Your Way Lean* plan.

Max: To raise your VO$_2$ max, which is the maximum amount of oxygen your body can use and the benchmark for good fitness, you need to take it to the max. These intervals are meant to be done full out as hard as you can—Zone 5, or a 9 to 10 on the RPE scale. The good news: Because they're so hard, they're also very short, lasting 20 seconds to 3 minutes.

Brisk: If VO$_2$ max is your roof, lactate threshold—the point at which you start working anaerobically—is the drop ceiling that hangs from it. Your goal is to raise your LT so you have a bigger aerobic room. There are lots of ways to train LT, including climbing hills and sustained efforts. These are done at an RPE of 7 to 8, Zone 4.

Steady: Also called tempo intervals, these efforts push you just above your comfort zone, so you're breathing faster and working harder than you would on a typical aerobic, endurance ride. But you're not working so hard that you can't sustain it for a long period of time. Steady efforts improve your body's ability to clear lactic acid, so they also help raise your LT. They're done at an RPE of 5 to 6, Zone 3.

Cruising: Let the good times roll. This is where you spend your long Sunday rides. This pleasant intensity is hard enough to feel like you're getting exercise, but you can carry on a conversation, cruise for hours, and enjoy the ride. These efforts build capillaries and endurance. Cruising rides are done at RPE 3 to 4, Zone 2.

Easy: For hard intervals to work their magic, you need easy rides and rest periods to let your body heal, adapt, and get stronger and fitter. Your easy days and recovery periods between intervals should be ridiculously easy—a pleasure ride that hovers in Zone 1, a 1 to 2 on the RPE scale.

Ramps: Occasionally, you'll find intervals called ramps. As the name implies, ramp intervals start in one of the lower zones and work up to a higher zone over a period of minutes. These are great for simulating real riding situations.

ADD MUSCLE INTO THE MIX

Strength-training is a critical piece of the puzzle for each plan. Making a little muscle increases your metabolism, strengthens your core to stabilize you on the bike for greater power and comfort on longer rides, boosts your confidence, and hey, makes you look good too. When possible, incorporate the *Ride Your Way Lean* strength plan 2 to 3 days weekly, on days that you are also performing specific intensity work (Tuesday, Thursday, and Saturday or Sunday). This may seem counterintuitive at first, but adding strength work on days when you should be resting, recovery riding, or cruising can interfere with your recovery and slow your regeneration. It's important to reserve those days for just that, recovery and adaptation from the previous day's load. Additionally, after performing specific work on the bike, your mind and body will be focused, amped up, and ready for more work. A quick 20-minute strength routine should be no problem at this point. Perform your strength routine following your bike workout, as this will allow you full energy to push the pedals, create cycling adaptations, and perform calorie-burning aerobic work. Your bike workout will also serve as a great warmup for your strength routine.

FUEL WISELY

There's an entire chapter (Chapter 5) on how to eat to ride, so we'll keep it short here. Studies show that exercise plus diet work better for long-term weight loss than either does alone. Recently, there's even been a bit of a backlash against exercise as a means of weight loss. Don't believe the hype. As any of the riders in this book (quite a few of whom have lost triple-digit weight) can tell you, exercise is essential for losing pounds and, more important, keeping them off. But they'll also tell you, all the riding in the world won't work if you have terrible eating habits.

Losing weight, no matter how little or how much you have to lose, takes patience, dedication, and workout intensity, while eating the right types of foods to keep your body fueled and your brain feeling fed and happy. Too many people focus on the task of cutting a particular macronutrient (protein, carbs, and fat) out of the diet as a quick pound-shedding fix. That may help you lose weight in the short term, but it's not sustainable and is certainly not good for your mind or your muscles.

As tempting as fad diets are—and they certainly are tempting when it seems like everyone is on them—steer clear of them, regardless of how promising they sound. Whether it's Atkins or the low-something diet of the month, it won't work long term. If it did, everyone would be on it, and we would have no more weight problems in this country. To be strong, happy, and lean, you need healthy doses of protein, carbohydrates, and fat. The following chapter will detail just how to fix your plate to get it done.

KEEP THE RESULTS COMING

Once you've completed your plan, it's important to evaluate your status to determine your next steps. For example, if you started at the Drop a Size or More plan but still have some stubborn pounds to shed, try moving on to the next plan (Shed the Stubborn Spare Tire). Spend the next 9 to 12 weeks finishing what you started. Did you achieve your weight-loss goals? If so, this is a great time to jump into the Fit for Life 12-week plan and continue the progression with your strength-training routine, shifting from beginner to intermediate, then advanced. For those who are ready to be fit for life, keep in mind the training concepts of overload, adaptation, and progression. Your body always needs to be challenged to keep from sliding backward. The Fit for Life plan will get you in the swing of riding and training (even if you're not racing) long term. When this 12-week plan comes to an end, I want you to feel confident about what's next.

This is where you'll need to take the structure you've developed and up the ante on the challenge and intensity as you adapt and get stronger, fitter, and faster. Realistically, most of us can only increase the volume (hours/miles) we ride by so much, because we simply run out of free time and daylight. That means your intensity and/or the amount of time you spend at a higher intensity will need to increase. As you complete your Fit for Life plan, you will be able to complete a 30-minute steady effort at a consistent pace. Let's say this pace is 18 mph, for example. Your strategy for increasing this steady pace is to try shorter intervals at 19 to 20 mph (3 × 10 minutes or 2 × 15 minutes at that pace), so that you are eventually able to duplicate the 30-minute effort at a higher speed and power output with the same level of exertion.

Continue with the structure of your plan, which labels Tuesday, Thursday, and Saturday as specific-intensity days, as you move forward. These days can be spent riding in target training ranges or riding with a group that will create a similar training stimulus. If the Tuesday, Thursday, Saturday structure is not conducive to your schedule, just be certain to take a rest, active recovery, or cruising-paced ride between specific-intensity sessions.

If you've come up a bit short on your weight-loss goals, don't be discouraged. Fair or not (not!), everyone burns calories and loses fat at different rates. And yes, there are some people for whom it just takes a little more time. So long as you're moving in the right direction, keep going.

On the following pages, you will find four exercise plans based on how much weight you want to lose. Each calendar block in the plan (see sample titled "Tuesday" on page 64) tells you what to do on each day. You'll find the total time for your prescribed ride in the top row; in this example, it's an hour. In the body of the block you'll find the type of ride you're to do. In this case, the ride is "Cruising+," or a Zone 2 endurance ride. You'll also find any intervals that are prescribed for the day. In this sample ride, below, you should include three 8-minute intervals at steady (or Zone 3) effort with 5 minutes' rest between intervals (RBI). If no RBI is prescribed, allow yourself to fully recover at a lower intensity between efforts. Pick your plan and let's get it started.

TUESDAY
1:00
Cruising+
3 x 8 min
Steady
5 min RBI

PLAN: BIG WEIGHT LOSS

Your long-term goal is to lose 35 to 50 pounds or more, with a short-term focus of 2 to 3 pounds per week. Your weekly targets might seem a bit aggressive, but for those with much to lose, the weight will come off quickly when following the proper recipe. Initially, you will shed weight at a more accelerated rate, tapering to smaller losses as you near your goal weight. Your primary keys to success are dedication and consistency. We'll spend the next 15 weeks riding 6 days weekly at varying intensities. The volume and intensity will build week by week. When you have the time, break free and extend your long rides. A nice, long, steady ride will definitely burn stored fat—and it's really fun. But I recognize that most of us just don't have that kind of time. Since higher intensity burns more calories, our focus will be on including a good number of steady- and brisk-intensity intervals designed to burn the fire a little hotter and tip the caloric scales in your favor.

While your training plan kicks off with relatively short hour-long rides during the week, it is always possible to add a bit of volume to any of the scheduled rides in your cruising range when your schedule permits. Just take care of yourself. It's easy to get excited and want to ride, ride, ride right out of the gate, especially when you have your goals set high. But respect your current level of fitness and don't drastically overdo it on any given day. If you're just coming off coach potato status, a 15- to 30-minute addition in workout time for any given ride is perfectly acceptable. If you've been riding consistently for a lengthy period of time before beginning your plan, a 30- to 60-minute addition to a workout is realistic.

For big weight loss to occur, big changes need to take place. You need to be honest with yourself about where those changes need to happen. Only you can pinpoint your weak link. You may be a consistent cyclist or exerciser who simply consumes too much junk food, oversized meals, or way too many calories late in the day. Conversely, you may eat a relatively healthy diet, but you've been riding the couch for so long, your metabolism has slowed, and your weight has gradually increased. Wherever your hurdles lie, be mindful of the challenge ahead and focus your energy in the appropriate places. Consistency in riding, good eating habits, and sometimes just pushing away from the table sooner will take you right where you want to go, confirms Pete Wingert, 41, of Kalispell, Montana.

"In April 2009, I weighed 245 pounds," recalls Pete, who at 6'7"still found that too much weight to bear. "I dug out my old mountain bike. I was barely able to ride it about 7 miles and went home defeated. I worked my way up to daily 20-plus-mile rides, with 30- to 40-mile rides on weekends. I continued to ride and bought a trainer in October. I currently weigh 205," says Pete, who credits consistency, patience, and intervals for his continued success. "I feel better than I have in 10 years and have lost 5 inches off my waistline. My BP has dropped too."

big weight loss

	MON	TUES	WED	THURS	FRI	SAT	SUN	WEEKLY TOTAL
Week 1	Rest Day	1:00	1:00	1:00	0:30	2:00	1:30	7:00
		Cruising+	Cruising	Cruising+	Easy	Cruising+	Cruising	
		3 x 8 min		4 x 5 min		3 x 10–12 min		
		Steady		Brisk		Steady Hills		
		5 min RBI		3 min RBI		Or Challenging Group Ride		

(continued)

	MON	TUES	WED	THURS	FRI	SAT	SUN	WEEKLY TOTAL
Week 2	Rest Day	1:00 Cruising+ 3 x 10 min Steady 5 min RBI	1:00 Cruising	1:00 Cruising+ 5 x 5 min Brisk 3 min RBI	0:30 Easy	2:00 Cruising+ 3 x 12–15 min Steady Hills Or Challenging Group Ride	1:30 Cruising	7:00
Week 3—Rest Week	Rest Day	1:00 Cruising	0:45 Cruising+ 3 x 5 min Steady 5 min RBI	1:00 Cruising	Rest Day	1:30 Cruising+ 2 x 10 min Steady Or Moderate Group Ride	1:00 Cruising	5:15
Week 4	Rest Day	1:15 Cruising+ 2 x 15 min Steady 5 min RBI	1:00 Cruising	1:00 Cruising+ 4 x 6 min Brisk 3 min RBI	0:35 Easy	2:15 Cruising+ 2 x 20 min Steady Hills Or Challenging Group Ride	1:45 Cruising	7:50
Week 5	Rest Day	1:15 Cruising+ 1 x 10 min Steady 3 x 6 min Brisk 3 min RBI	1:00 Cruising	1:00 Cruising+ 1 x 15 min Steady 3 x 5 min Brisk 3 min RBI	0:35 Easy	2:15 Cruising+ 1 x 20 min Steady 2 x 10 min Brisk Or Challenging Group Ride	1:45 Cruising	7:50
Week 6	Rest Day	1:00 Cruising	0:45 Cruising+ 3 x 5 min Steady	1:00 Cruising	Rest Day	1:30 Cruising+ 3 x 10 min Steady	1:00 Cruising	5:15

	MON	TUES	WED	THURS	FRI	SAT	SUN	WEEKLY TOTAL
Rest Week			5 min RBI			Or Moderate Group Ride		
Week 7	Rest Day	1:15	1:15	1:15	0:40	2:15	2:00	8:40
		Cruising+	Cruising	Cruising+	Easy	Cruising+	Cruising	
		1 x 20 min		2 x 10 min		3 x 15 min Ramps		
		Steady		Brisk		8 min Steady, 5 min Brisk, 2 min Max		
		3 x 1 min		3 x 1 min		8–10 min RBI		
		Max		Max		Or Group Ride		
		2 min RBI		2 min RBI				
Week 8	Rest Day	1:15	1:15	1:15	0:40	2:15	2:00	8:40
		Cruising+	Cruising	Cruising+	Easy	Cruising+	Cruising	
		1 x 20 min		2 x 12 min		3 x 15 min Ramps		
		Steady		Brisk		6 min Steady, 7 min Brisk, 2 min Max		
		4 x 1 min		4 x 1 min		8–10 min RBI		
		Max		Max		Or Group Ride		
		90 sec RBI		90 sec RBI				
Week 9—Rest Week	Rest Day	1:00	1:00	1:00	Rest Day	1:30	1:15	5:45
		Cruising	Cruising+	Cruising		Cruising+	Cruising	
			4 x 5 min			3 x 15 min		
			Steady			Steady		
			5 min RBI			Or Moderate Group Ride		
Week 10	Rest Day	1:15	1:15	1:15	0:45	2:30	2:00	9:00
		Cruising+	Cruising	Cruising+	Easy	Cruising+	Cruising	
		1 x 25 min		2 x 12 min		3 x 15 min Ramps		

(continued)

	MON	TUES	WED	THURS	FRI	SAT	SUN	WEEKLY TOTAL
Week 10		Steady		Brisk		5 min Steady, 8 min Brisk, 2 min Max		
		3 x 90 sec		6 min RBI		8 min RBI		
		Max		3 x 90 sec		Or Challenging Group Ride		
		2 min RBI		Max				
				2 min RBI				
Week 11	Rest Day	1:15	1:15	1:15	0:45	2:30	2:00	9:00
		Cruising+	Cruising	Cruising+	Easy	Cruising+	Cruising	
		1 x 10 min		1 x 15 min		3 x 15 min		
		Steady		Brisk		Brisk Hills		
		5 x 5 min		4 x 90 sec		4 x 10 sec		
		Brisk		Max		Sprints		
		2 min RBI		2 min RBI		Or Group Ride		
Week 12 — Rest Week	Rest Day	1:00	1:15	1:00	Rest Day	1:45	1:15	6:15
		Cruising	Cruising+	Cruising		Cruising+	Cruising	
			4 x 5 min			3 x 15 min		
			Steady			Steady		
			5 min RBI			Or Moderate Group Ride		
Week 13	Rest Day	1:15	1:30	1:15	1:00	2:45	2:15	10:00
		Cruising+	Cruising	Cruising+	Easy	Cruising+	Cruising	
		1 x 15 min		1 x 20 min		2 x 20 min		
		Steady		Brisk		Brisk Hills		
		4 x 5 min		3 x 2 min		5 x 10 sec		
		4 min Brisk, 1 min Max		Max		Sprints		
		3 min RBI		2 min RBI		Or Group Ride		
Week 14	Rest Day	1:15	1:30	1:15	1:00	2:45	2:15	10:00
		Cruising+	Cruising	Cruising+	Easy	Cruising+	Cruising	
		1 x 20 min		2 x 15 min		2 x 20 min		

	MON	TUES	WED	THURS	FRI	SAT	SUN	WEEKLY TOTAL
Week 14		Steady		Brisk		Brisk Hills		
		4 x 6 min		8 min RBI		4 x 2 min		
		4 min Brisk, 2 min Max		3 x 2 min		Max		
		3 min RBI		Max		2 min RBI		
				90 sec RBI		Or Group Ride		
Week 15— Rest Week	Rest Day	1:00	1:15	1:00	Rest Day	1:45	1:30	6:30
		Cruising	Cruising+	Cruising		Cruising+	Cruising	
			5 x 5 min			3 x 15 min		
			Steady			Steady		
			5 min RBI			Or Moderate Group Ride		

✳DROP A SIZE OR MORE

Dropping a size or more, 15- to 35-pound weight loss, is a formidable goal, but one that you can achieve with a bit of hard work. Your short-term target is 1.5 to 3 pounds weekly. Your 12-week plan was designed with a primary focus on steady and brisk pace work peppered with higher intensity max intervals and sprints. The hotter you burn the fire, the more calories you'll burn and the more fitness you'll gain. Focused interval work that takes you out of your comfort zone is your key for taking control. Too many cyclists are content riding at a moderately challenging aerobic pace, but not one that truly pushes their limits, burns excess calories and body weight, or creates tremendous fitness gains. For those with weight-loss goals, it is mission critical to step it up and push yourself like you've never pushed before. I've coached plenty of athletes who train 6 days a week but can't seem to shed extra body weight. The day they decide to let go of their endless comfort-zone riding and step on the gas, they enjoy a nearly miraculous transformation. Yes, it's a bit painful at first, but you'll grow to enjoy it and it pays big dividends.

15 - 35 lbs

RIDE YOUR WAY LEAN

drop a size or more

	MON	TUES	WED	THURS	FRI	SAT	SUN	WEEKLY TOTAL
Week 1	Rest Day	1:00	1:15	1:00	0:30	2:00	1:30	7:15
		Cruising+	Cruising	Cruising+	Easy	Cruising+	Cruising	
		1 x 10 min		3 x 10 min		3 x 8 min		
		Steady		Steady		Hills (2 Steady, 1 Brisk)		
		3 x 5 min		5 min RBI		Or Challenging Group Ride		
		Brisk Hills or Flats		Finish each w/ 30 sec Max				
		5 min RBI						
Week 2	Rest Day	1:00	1:15	1:00	0:30	2:00	1:30	7:15
		Cruising+	Cruising	Cruising+	Easy	Cruising+	Cruising	
		2 x 10 min		3 x 5 min		3 x 10 min		
		Steady		Brisk		Hills (2 Steady, 1 Brisk)		
		1 x 10 min		3 min RBI		Or Challenging Group Ride		
		Brisk		4 x 10 sec				
		5 min RBI		Sprints				
				5 min RBI				
Week 3 — Rest Week	Rest Day	1:00	0:45	1:00	Rest Day	1:30	1:00	5:15
		Cruising	Cruising+	Cruising		Cruising+	Cruising	
			1 x 5 min			3 x 6 min		
			Steady			Steady		
			2 x 3 min			Or Moderate Group Ride		
			Brisk					
			5 min RBI					
Week 4	Rest Day	1:00	1:15	1:00	0:40	2:15	1:30	7:40
		Cruising+	Cruising	Cruising+	Easy	Cruising+	Cruising	
		3 x 10 min		1 x 10 min		3 x 10 min		

	MON	TUES	WED	THURS	FRI	SAT	SUN	WEEKLY TOTAL
Week 4		Steady		Brisk		Hills (1 Steady, 2 Brisk)		
		8 min RBI		5 x 30 sec		Or Challenging Group Ride		
				Max				
				3 min RBI				
Week 5	Rest Day	1:15	1:00	1:15	0:40	2:15	1:45	8:10
		Cruising+	Cruising	Cruising+	Easy	Cruising+	Cruising	
		5 x 5 min		1 x 20 min		3 x 10 min		
		Brisk		Steady		Brisk Hills		
		3 min RBI		4 x 4 min		Or Challenging Group Ride		
		1 x 15 min		Brisk				
		Steady		2 min RBI				
Week 6— Rest Week	Rest Day	1:00	0:45	1:00	Rest Day	1:30	1:15	5:30
		Cruising	Cruising+	Cruising		Cruising+	Cruising	
			1 x 5 min			2 x 10 min		
			Steady			Steady		
			3 x 3 min			Or Moderate Group Ride		
			Brisk					
			5 min RBI					
Week 7	Rest Day	1:15	1:00	1:15	0:45	2:30	1:45	8:30
		Cruising+	Cruising	Cruising+	Easy	Cruising+	Cruising	
		2 x 15 min		3 x 12 min Ramps		3 x 12 min		
		Steady		6 min Steady, 5 min Brisk, 1 min Max		Brisk Hills		
		10 min RBI		8 min RBI		Or Challenging Group Ride		

(continued)

	MON	TUES	WED	THURS	FRI	SAT	SUN	WEEKLY TOTAL
Week 7		3 x 1 min						
		Max						
		3 min RBI						
Week 8	Rest Day	1:15	1:00	1:15	0:45	2:30	1:45	8:30
		Cruising+	Cruising	Cruising+	Easy	Cruising+	Cruising	
		3 x 10 min		1 x 20 min		4 x 10 min		
		Brisk		Steady		Brisk Hills		
		5 min RBI		4 x 1 min		Or Challenging Group Ride		
		3 x 30 sec		Max				
		Max						
		1 min RBI		3 min RBI				
Week 9— Rest Week	Rest Day	1:00	1:00	1:00	0:30	1:30	1:15	6:15
		Cruising	Cruising+	Cruising	Easy	Cruising+	Cruising	
			2 x 5 min			3 x 8 min		
			Steady			Steady		
			2 x 5 min			Or Moderate Group Ride		
			Brisk					
			5 min RBI					
Week 10	Rest Day	1:15	1:00	1:15	0:45	2:45	1:45	8:45
		Cruising+	Cruising	Cruising+	Easy	Cruising+	Cruising	
		1 x 20 min		1 x 20 min		3 x 15 min		
		Steady		Steady		Brisk Hills		
		4 x 90 sec		1 x 15 min		Or Challenging Group Ride		
		Max		Brisk				
		3 min RBI		10 min RBI				
Week 11	Rest Day	1:15	1:00	1:30	0:45	2:45	2:00	9:15
		Cruising+	Cruising	Cruising+	Easy	Cruising+	Cruising	
		2 x 15 min		3 x 15 min Ramps		2 x 20–25 min		

	MON	TUES	WED	THURS	FRI	SAT	SUN	WEEKLY TOTAL
Week 11		Brisk		5 min Steady, 9 min Brisk, 1 min Max		Brisk Hills		
		10 min RBI		10 min RBI		Or Challenging Group Ride		
		4 x 90 sec						
		Max						
		2 min RBI						
Week 12—Rest Week	Rest Day	1:00	1:00	1:00	0:45	1:30	1:30	6:45
		Cruising	Cruising+	Cruising	Easy	Cruising+	Cruising	
			2 x 5 min			3 x 10 min		
			Steady			Steady		
			2 x 5 min			Or Moderate Group Ride		
			Brisk					
			3 min RBI					

✳SHED THE STUBBORN SPARE TIRE

You're not far from your goal; 5 to 15 pounds is just around the corner, a mere 9 weeks ahead. Your short-term goal is a target of 0.5 to 1.5 pounds weekly. Shedding that stubborn spare tire is a simple function of tightening the screws on your diet and exercise. A collage of intervals that include steady, brisk, and max efforts makes up your plan. Stepping into those higher intensity ranges will burn extra calories in a short period of time while improving your fitness along the way.

You may have been spending a bit too much time in that comfort zone or put on a few holiday pounds that just never came off. Maybe you had a baby, got caught up in career, or just got carried away with late nights and eating out. Whatever the case, it's time to focus and turn up the heat. Consistency with riding, the added intensity, and trimming the fluff from your diet should bring you back in line.

One quick way to bring your eating back into control is a food log. Record everything you eat and drink for a 3-day period. Include the approximate amount of food and the time of day it was consumed. Once you see things in black and white, it becomes pretty apparent where the problem areas lie. Check for small things you can eliminate that serve no nutritional purpose: candy, pastries, sodas, high-calorie condiments like cream dressings or sauces. Are you eating too much processed food or overly large meals or doing a lot of late-night snacking? Use your dietary recall to identify the areas of concern and plan your attack accordingly.

shed the stubborn spare tire

	MON	TUES	WED	THURS	FRI	SAT	SUN	WEEKLY TOTAL
Week 1	Rest Day	1:00	1:00	1:00	0:30	1:30	1:30	6:30
		Cruising+	Cruising+	Cruising	Easy	Cruising+	Cruising+	
		1 x 10 min	3 x 10 min			2 x 30 min	2 x 15 min	
		Brisk	Steady			10 min Steady, 10 min Brisk, 10 min Steady	Brisk	
		5 x 1 min	5 min RBI				10 min RBI	
		Max	5 x 30 sec				4 x 90 sec	
		3 min RBI	Max				Max	
			1 min RBI				3 min RBI	
Week 2	Rest Day	1:00	1:00	1:00	0:30	2:00	1:30	7:00
		Cruising+	Cruising+	Cruising	Easy	Cruising+	Cruising+	
		1 x 12 min	2 x 15 min			2 x 35 min	1 x 20 min	
		Brisk	Steady			10 min Steady, 15 min Brisk, 10 min Steady	Brisk	

	MON	TUES	WED	THURS	FRI	SAT	SUN	WEEKLY TOTAL
Week 2		4 x 90 sec	5 min RBI				10 min RBI	
		Max	6 x 30 sec				5 x 90 sec	
		3 min RBI	Max				Max	
			1 min RBI				3 min RBI	
Week 3— Rest Week	Rest Day	1:00	0:45	1:00	0:30	1:30	1:00	5:45
		Cruising	Cruising+	Cruising	Easy	Cruising+	Cruising	
			2 x 10 min			1 x 15 min		
			Steady			Steady		
			10 min RBI			2 x 5 min		
						Brisk		
						10 min RBI		
Week 4	Rest Day	1:15	1:00	1:00	0:30	2:00	1:45	7:30
		Cruising+	Cruising+	Cruising	Easy	Cruising+	Cruising+	
		1 x 15 min	1 x 15 min			2 x 20 min Ramps	3 x 10 min	
		Brisk	Steady			10 min Steady, 8 min Brisk, 2 min Max	Brisk Hills	
		5 x 90 sec	1 x 10 min			10 min RBI	5–8 min RBI	
		Max	Brisk					
		2 min RBI	6 x 30 sec					
			Max					
			1 min RBI					
Week 5	Rest Day	1:15	1:00	1:00	0:45	2:15	1:45	8:00
		Cruising+	Cruising+	Cruising	Easy	Cruising+	Cruising	
		1 x 20 min	1 x 30 min			2 x 25 min Ramps		

(continued)

	MON	TUES	WED	THURS	FRI	SAT	SUN	WEEKLY TOTAL
Week 5		Brisk	Steady			12 min Steady, 10 min Brisk, 3 min Max		
		5 x 90 sec	5 x 30 sec			15 min RBI		
		Max	Max					
		90 sec RBI	30 sec RBI					
Week 6 — Rest Week	Rest Day	1:00	0:45	1:00	0:30	1:30	1:00	5:45
		Cruising	Cruising+	Cruising	Easy	Cruising+	Cruising	
			1 x 20 min			1 x 10 min		
			Steady			Steady		
						1 x 10 min		
						Brisk		
Week 7	Rest Day	1:15	1:00	1:15	0:45	2:30	1:45	8:30
		Cruising+	Cruising+	Cruising	Easy	Cruising+	Cruising	
		1 x 20 min	1 x 30 min			3 x 15 min		
		Brisk	Steady			Steady Hills		
		5 x 10 sec	5 x 1 min			2 x 10 min		
		Sprints	Max			Brisk Flats		
		5 min RBI	2 min RBI					
Week 8	Rest Day	1:15	1:00	1:15	1:00	2:30	2:00	9:00
		Cruising+	Cruising+	Cruising	Easy	Cruising+	Cruising	
		1 x 25 min	1 x 30 min			3 x 20 min		
		Brisk	Steady			Steady Hills		
		5 x 10 sec	4 x 2 min			5 x 10 sec		

	MON	TUES	WED	THURS	FRI	SAT	SUN	WEEKLY TOTAL
Week 8		Sprints	Max			Sprints		
		5 min RBI	2 min RBI			5 min RBI		
Week 9—Rest Week	Rest Day	1:00	0:45	1:00	0:45	1:30	1:00	6:00
		Cruising	Cruising+	Cruising	Easy	Cruising+	Cruising	
			4 x 10 sec			1 x 20 min		
			Sprints			Steady		
			5 min RBI			4 x 10 sec		
						Sprints		

✳FIT FOR LIFE

Congratulations! You've finally arrived. You've hit your weight-loss goals and are ready to stay fit for life. This 12-week plan will provide variety, fun, and sound guidance as you step forward on your journey. The two keys to lifelong fitness are variety and overload. You must keep your riding new and fresh in order to keep the motivation high for spinning your wheels. Granted, sometimes it feels like you're doing the same five rides with the same three friends week in and week out. But don't let that wear on you, nor should it become the norm. Challenge yourself to seek out new routes, riding partners, clubs, events, and other cycling disciplines (mountain, track, cyclocross). Variety and new challenges will keep your motivation high.

One pitfall I'd caution you against—and one that I've seen many a rider fall into—is becoming a "maintenance exerciser." There's no quicker way to lose fitness, and watch some of that weight creep back on, than to decide that it's time to skate. When James Herrera poses the question, "Would you classify yourself as a maintenance exerciser?" to audiences around the country, about 75 percent of the hands shoot up into the air, he says. Sure, it seems like a logical thing. You're not training for a race or particular event per se, just riding for enjoyment, stress relief, camaraderie, and fitness, right? The problem with the maintenance label is, it oftentimes gives cyclists a license to stagnate in their performance. "If I'm maintaining, I don't need to go any harder than I am now." Wrong.

Maintenance is a function of perceived exertion and metabolic work, but we *always* want to progressively overload ourselves so we continue to gain fitness. More simply put, if my heart is working at 140 beats per minute while I travel 16-mph, a good form of maintenance is to increase my pace to 18 mph while still working at 140 bpm. My perceived exertion is the same, my metabolic work is the same, but my pace has increased. A false form of maintenance exercising, which is what I see most people do, is to keep focusing on that initial 16-mph pace. Riders will lose fitness over time due to a failure to challenge themselves with moderate overloads. In short, you run the risk of backsliding if you try riding to stay in the same place.

The take-home message as you move ahead with your fitness for life plan is to constantly push yourself with higher-intensity efforts, challenging group rides, and variety in your routes, groups, and bikes. Mind you, this doesn't mean that *every* ride is a hammerfest. You won't help yourself by going hard all the time either. Just keep doing what you did to help you get to where you are: Work hard sometimes, recover others, and step up to new challenges along the way. At some point, you'll find that your goals for and benefits from cycling transcend weight loss, as in the case of John Rockwell, 37, from Moreno Valley, California, who began cycling last summer to lose weight and after riding 20 to 40 miles most days lost 50 pounds.

"The weight is not so much the focus anymore. Seeing my little corner of the world from the seat of my LeMond has helped me to appreciate the thousands of miles of beautiful Southern California scenery out there," he says wistfully. "I see how much I took for granted, and gained a new perspective. I actually like where I live now. I am inspired to go exercise, and I spend a heck of a lot more mental energy looking forward to a 20- to 40-mile ride each day than I do wondering how much weight I might lose in a given week." Sounds like John is truly fit for life.

fit for life

	MON	TUES	WED	THURS	FRI	SAT	SUN
Week 1	Rest Day	1:00–1:15	1:00–1:30	1:00–1:15	0:30–0:45	1:30–2:30	1:30–2:00
		Cruising+	Cruising	Cruising+	Easy	Challenging Group/Fun Ride	Cruising+
		30 min	Or Moderate Group/Fun Ride	30 min	Or Rest Day		3 x 15 min
		Steady		Brisk			Steady Hills
							Or Moderate Group/Fun Ride
Week 2	Rest Day	1:00–1:15	1:00–1:30	1:00–1:15	0:30–0:45	1:30–2:30	1:30–2:00
		Cruising+	Cruising	Cruising+	Easy	Challenging Group/Fun Ride	Cruising+
		35 min	Or Moderate Group/Fun Ride	35 min	Or Rest Day		2 x 20 min
		Steady		Brisk			Steady Hills
							Or Moderate Group/Fun Ride
Week 3	Rest Day	1:00	0:45–1:15	1:00	Rest Day	1:30–2:00	1:15–1:30
		Cruising	Cruising	Cruising		Moderate to Light Group/Fun Ride	Cruising

(continued)

	MON	TUES	WED	THURS	FRI	SAT	SUN
Rest Week			Or Light Group/Fun Ride				Or Moderate Pace Fun Ride
Week 4	Rest Day	1:00–1:30	1:00–1:30	1:00–1:30	0:30–0:45	1:45–2:45	1:30–2:15
		Cruising+	Cruising	Cruising+	Easy	Challenging Group/Fun Ride	Cruising+
		40 min	Or Moderate Group/Fun Ride	40 min	Or Rest Day		1 x 20 min
		Steady		Brisk			Steady
							2 x 15 min
							Brisk
							Or Challenging Group/Fun Ride
Week 5	Rest Day	1:00–130	1:00–1:30	1:00–1:30	0:30–0:45	1:45–2:45	1:30–2:15
		Cruising+	Cruising	Cruising+	Easy	Challenging Group/Fun Ride	Cruising+
		45 min	Or Moderate Group/Fun Ride	45 min	Or Rest Day		1 x 15 min
		Steady		Brisk			Steady
							2 x 20 min
							Brisk
							Or Challenging Group/Fun Ride
Week 6	Rest Day	1:00–1:15	0:45–1:15	1:00–1:15	Rest Day	1:30–2:00	1:15–1:30
		Cruising	Cruising	Cruising		Moderate to Light Group/Fun Ride	Cruising

	MON	TUES	WED	THURS	FRI	SAT	SUN
Rest Week			Or Light Group/Fun Ride				Or Moderate Pace Fun Ride
Week 7	Rest Day	1:00–1:30	1:00–1:30	1:00–1:30	0:30–1:00	1:45–3:00	1:30–2:30
		Cruising+	Cruising	Cruising+	Easy	Challenging Group/Fun Ride	Cruising+
		20 min Steady	Or Moderate Group/Fun Ride	20 min Steady	Or Rest Day		3 x 15 min
		20 min		20 min			Brisk Hills
		Brisk		Brisk			Or Challenging Group/Fun Ride
		3 x 10 sec		3 x 10 sec			
		Sprints		Sprints			
Week 8	Rest Day	1:00–1:30	1:00–1:30	1:00–1:30	0:30–1:00	1:45–3:00	1:30–2:30
		Cruising+	Cruising	Cruising+	Easy	Challenging Group/Fun Ride	Cruising+
		25 min	Or Moderate Group/Fun Ride	20 min	Or Rest Day		3 x 15 min Ramps
		Steady		Steady			5 min Steady, 8 min Brisk, 2 min Max
		20 min		25 min			Or Challenging Group/Fun Ride
		Brisk		Brisk			
		3 x 10 sec		3 x 10 sec			
		Sprints		Sprints			

(continued)

	MON	TUES	WED	THURS	FRI	SAT	SUN
Week 9—Rest Week	Rest Day	1:00–1:15	0:45–1:15	1:00–1:15	Rest Day	1:30–2:00	1:15–1:30
		Cruising	Cruising	Cruising		Moderate to Light Group/Fun Ride	Cruising
			Or Light Group/Fun Ride				Or Moderate Pace Fun Ride
Week 10	Rest Day	1:00–1:30	1:00–1:30	1:00–1:30	0:30–1:00	1:45–3:00	1:30–2:45
		Cruising+	Cruising	Cruising+	Easy	Challenging Group/Fun Ride	Cruising+
		30 min	Or Moderate Group/Fun Ride	15 min	Or Rest Day		3 x 18 min Ramps
		Steady		Steady			8 min Steady, 8 min Brisk, 2 min Max
		15 min		30 min			Or Challenging Group/Fun Ride
		Brisk		Brisk			
		4 x 10 sec		4 x 10 sec			
		Sprints		Sprints			
Week 11	Rest Day	1:00–1:30	1:00–1:30	1:00–1:30	0:30–1:00	1:45–3:00	1:30–2:45
		Cruising+	Cruising	Cruising+	Easy	Challenging Group/Fun Ride	Cruising+
		20 min	Or Moderate Group/Fun Ride	15 min	Or Rest Day		3 x 20 min Ramps
		Steady		Steady			10 min Steady, 8 min Brisk, 2 min Max

	MON	TUES	WED	THURS	FRI	SAT	SUN
Week 11		15 min		20 min			Or Challenging Group/Fun Ride
		Brisk		Brisk			
		3 x 1 min		5 x 1 min			
		Max		Max			
Week 12— Rest Week	Rest Day	1:00–1:15	0:45–1:15	1:00–1:15	Rest Day	1:30–2:00	1:15–1:30
		Cruising	Cruising	Cruising		Moderate to Light Group/Fun Ride	Cruising
			Or Light Group/Fun Ride				Or Moderate Pace Fun Ride

5: EAT TO LOSE

EAT TO RIDE. RIDE TO EAT. SHED POUNDS BY DOING BOTH

ET'S FACE IT, getting off the sofa and onto your bike will help you peel off pounds. But when we pile them on, it's generally not just lack of exercise that's to blame. It's also how much— and how much of what—we eat that does us in. Little wonder. Not only do we live in a culture that's rife with calorie pollution, but also most of us are woefully in the dark when it comes to understanding exactly what we need to eat.

According to a recent survey by the International Food Information Council Foundation, more than three-quarters of Americans still don't know good fats from bad fats; only 15 percent of us know about how many calories we should eat every day; and despite the constant drilling of the "most important meal of the day message," fewer than half of us eat breakfast every morning. Given our general dearth of nutritional knowledge, it's no great surprise that more than two-thirds of us are now overweight.

To be brutally honest, sometimes we're to blame. We know our eating is off the rails, but we just can't manage to take the first step to fix it. That was the case with Yuri Polyak, a 42-year-old triathlete who once weighed over 300 pounds. Like so many overweight adults, he got away with murderously poor eating habits when he was young by playing sports—football and swimming, in his case. But once in the realm of "real life," the old, unchecked eating habits came home to roost, and roost some more in the form of stored fat and unwanted pounds.

"I really had no idea about nutrition," says Yuri. "I ate pizza, burgers, pasta, chips, ice cream, whatever I wanted at all hours of the day. I would skip meals and pay no attention to portion control. During those times when I did decide to lose weight, I would starve myself or go on a special diet, like Atkins. I'd always lose a bunch of weight. Then I'd fall back into my old habits and gain it all back with some extra pounds, because I'd end up bingeing on all the foods I'd deprived myself of." It wasn't until Yuri, who started cycling right before his 40th birthday, educated himself on the impact that fat, protein, and carbs had on his health and his riding that he made real, lasting modifications and finally dropped the weight for good.

"Now I eat fruits and vegetables; fish, chicken, and bison; whole grains; and dried fruit and nuts," says Yuri, who now weighs about 200 pounds. "I've learned how to eat before and after my workouts so I'm not starving all day. My whole diet has changed for the better. And so have I."

✳BACK TO BASICS

Though sometimes our overindulgences are of our own doing, just as often, we're a bit less to blame. It's confusing out there. I've been a health and science writer for 20 years. I've been a trainer for 15. In that time, I've seen low-fat and high-carb rise and fall in spectacular fashion—and I'm talking about official government recommendations à la the food pyramid. That's not even mentioning nutritional debacles known as "diets" that would have you believing it's ok to subsist on cabbage, raw foods, and liquid shakes in lieu of balanced meals.

There's plenty of disagreement even among seasoned (and successful) athletes, coaches, and sports nutritionists. James Herrera, who developed this book's weight-loss plan, is an avowed vegan. I was a longtime vegetarian but now eat meat and generally follow the Paleo philosophy of filling up on lean protein, vegetables, fruits, and unprocessed foods. Yet we agree 100 percent on how athletes should eat. How's that? Because though there are literally dozens of different dietary recommendations for optimum health and sports performance, if you line them up and examine them closely, you'll see that for all of their differences, they mostly agree on the same basic principles: Eat real, recognizable food; fill your plate with vegetables and fruits; choose your protein, carbs, and fats wisely; use food as fuel; and enjoy your food. Here's how.

CREATE A BALANCED PLATE

The biggest, fattest lie the nutrition industry (along with hundreds of other industries) has ever sold us is this notion that it doesn't matter whether you eat 3,500 extra calories from steamed broccoli or from sticky buns, you'll gain a pound either way because a calorie is a calorie is a calorie. Yes, a calorie is simply a measure of energy in food. But where those calories come from has a tremendous impact on how they're processed, burned, and stored. In the words of Cynthia Sass, MPH, RD, CSSD, a New York City–based sports nutritionist, "You get your calories from three basic sources: carbohydrates, protein, and fat. These macronutrients keep your body running the same way gasoline, motor oil, and essential fluids keep your car running. Your body processes them just as differently."

The effect of eating the right calorie combination is so profound that Sass says she's seen clients eat the perfect number of calories, but from the wrong sources, which resulted in not losing weight or, worse, gaining some. "This is especially true when clients cut their fat intake way too low," she says. "They don't have enough fat in their system, so the jobs that fat does, like repairing cell membranes and optimizing hormones, go undone and the surplus carbs they're eating instead get stored as fat. I've had numerous clients lose weight, improve their immune system, gain muscle, and boost energy by correcting the balance of carbs, protein, and fats, without changing their calorie intake."

What does that right balance look like? As you would expect, it looks *balanced,* with all macronutrients represented at every meal. Sass recommends aiming for 50 to 55 percent of your calories from carbs (think: fill half your plate with vegetables, fruits, and some whole grains), 25 to 30 percent from fat (olive oil, avocado, etc.), and 15 to 20 percent from protein (lean meats, fish, eggs, and poultry). That carbohydrate recommendation is lower than you'll see in many sports nutrition circles. But as your body becomes a better fat burner, you'll be able to ride well at this level. "Just be sure to skew your pre-workout meals or snacks to be heavier in carbs and lower in fat and protein to fuel up properly and avoid cramps," says Sass.

To create perfectly balanced meals, Sass suggests fruit, vegetable, and protein combinations like these from *The Flat Belly Diet*, which Sass coauthored:

Sweet and Sour Shrimp

$1/2$ teaspoon olive oil

8 ounces bell pepper strips

$1/3$ cup apricot jam

2 teaspoons red wine vinegar

6 ounces (1 cup) cooked, peeled, and deveined shrimp

$1/2$ cup chopped unsalted dry-roasted peanuts

Heat the oil in a nonstick skillet over medium-high heat. Add the peppers and cook, tossing, for about 3 minutes or until hot. Add the jam and vinegar. Cook for 1 minute, or until bubbling.

Add the shrimp and cook for 2 minutes, or until bubbling. Divide evenly onto 2 plates, and sprinkle with the peanuts.

Makes 2 servings.
Per serving: 357 calories, 23 grams protein, 44 grams carbohydrates, 11 grams fat.

Chicken with Banana Chutney Topping

7 ounces boneless, skinless cooked chicken breasts or cooked chicken pieces or canned chicken

$^1/_2$ medium banana, chopped

2 teaspoons mango chutney

$^1/_4$ cup toasted chopped cashews

$^1/_2$ teaspoon freshly squeezed lemon juice (about $^1/_2$ lemon)

Cut the chicken breasts into thin diagonal slices. Fan the slices out on 2 salad plates. If using precooked chicken, cut into bite-size pieces. If using canned chicken, crumble into bite-size pieces.

In a small bowl, combine the banana, chutney, cashews, and lemon juice. Stir gently to mix. Spoon over the chicken.

Makes 2 servings.
Per serving: 337 calories, 34 grams protein, 24 grams carbohydrates, 11.5 grams fat.

EAT ACTIVE CALORIES

Beyond eating the right balance of macronutrients is choosing more "active" calories. Certain calories make you work more to burn them, so you literally use more energy in the eating and digesting process. I call them "active" calories. On the other end of the spectrum are what I deem couch potato calories, those that come in foods that are so heavily processed they're nearly predigested. How much of each you eat can have a profound effect on your weight-loss success . . . or lack thereof. Leslie Bonci, MPH, RD, director of sports nutrition at University of Pittsburgh Medical Center, says that the preponderance of couch potato calories is partly to blame for our current obesity epidemic.

"That fast-food burger or chicken sandwich has gone through so much processing and pulverization, you barely have to chew," she says. "We're losing the ability to burn calories as we naturally would during the eating and digestive process." The solution: eat foods that are close to their natural state, such as fresh vegetables; fruits; lean, whole cuts of meat; legumes; nuts and seeds; and whole grains. "These foods require action—energy— from your body. You need to work to chew them and to digest them. They create what is known as a thermic response, which means you burn more calories just processing them." As you may have already guessed, these foods also tend to be far less energy dense (yet far more nutrient dense) than their lazy-calorie counterparts. They also tend to be rich in fiber and high in water content, so they fill you up faster and sustain you longer than highly processed foods.

Like Sass, Bonci doesn't recommend counting calories or calculating macronutrient grams and percentages, but rather changing the composition of your plate. By setting up a high-performance, active-calorie plate, you can lose weight without worrying about walking around hungry or bonking on your bike. It's easy and very similar to the balanced-plate recommendations on page 86. Simply fill one-half with active calories from fruits and vegetables. Fill one-quarter to one-third with active to semiactive calories (see chart) from protein such as lean meat, poultry, fish, soy foods, eggs, and low-fat dairy. Fill the other quarter with active and semiactive calories from whole-grain starches like brown rice, sweet potatoes, and whole-grain bread. You don't need to eliminate couch potato calories. Just eat them sparingly, mostly for occasional indulgences and snacks.

ACTIVE CALORIES	SEMIACTIVE CALORIES	COUCH POTATO CALORIES
Fruits	Whole-grain bread	Fast-food burgers, fries, and processed sandwiches
Vegetables	Fiber-rich cereal	Processed meats (i.e., bologna)
Whole grains	Whole-wheat pasta	Chips, pretzels, packaged snack foods
Beans and legumes	Low-fat dairy	Pastries, cookies, pies, and cakes
Lean meat, fish, poultry	Hearty soups	

✳BE CHOOSY WITH CARBS

Somewhere along the line, starchy foods like pasta, bread, and rice became synonymous with carbs. While spaghetti and bagels are indeed carbohydrates, and you do need carbohydrates for fuel, they're not the only source of energy for your working muscles, especially if you're trying to lose weight. Starchy carbs are as easy to overeat as potato chips (which are just fried starchy carbs), and any surplus gets socked away in your fat stores. "Your brain operates on sugar," explains exercise scientist Joe Friel, head coach at TrainingBible Coaching, and coauthor of *The Paleo Diet for Athletes*. "When you eat bagels and potatoes, your body turns them into sugar and delivers them to your cells very quickly, which makes your brain happy and leaves you wanting more." That's why it's hard to stop yourself from plowing through a basket of sourdough bread or a bowl of pasta. Starch has an addictive property that leaves you craving more food, but not because you're hungry.

Though you need some carbs to keep your glycogen stores stocked, don't make the mistake of thinking that all the carbs you eat will be neatly tucked into your muscle glycogen stores. Remember that your body can store only about 90 minutes' worth of glycogen-based energy in your muscles and liver. Once those stores are fully stocked, anything left over is ferried into long-term storage—in the form of fat.

That's why wise weight-conscious cyclists swap much of their starch for fruits and vegetables, especially when they're not on their bikes putting in big miles. These plant foods are rich in carbohydrates, but tend to be much lower in calories and digest far more slowly. When you focus on these foods, weight loss is almost effortless because you're far less likely to eat so many pears, bananas, tomatoes, and Brussels sprouts or so much spinach and broccoli that you end up with more calories than you need. (You can't really say the same about candy bars, white bread, and white rice, can you?) What's more, plant foods are brimming with vitamins, minerals, and immunity-building, free-radical-fighting antioxidants that make you healthier and stronger, so you can ride better and burn even more calories.

That's not to say you need to completely kiss your beloved bread and noodles good-bye. When you need quick-digesting carbs that shoot into your bloodstream fast and are ready for action, starchy carbs answer the call. In fact, I've found that if I save the starchy carbs for before, during, and after a hard, long ride or race, they work like rocket fuel, because my muscles are getting them exactly when they need them.

Also resist the temptation to cut too far back on carbs, cautions our diet plan guru, Performance Driven's James Herrera, who counsels athletes of all levels around the world. "They're your primary fuel source for sustainable energy when you're working hard. They're also the primary fuel source for your brain and other vital organs. Eliminating carbs—which some over-zealous athletes try to do—does nothing but cause distress, low energy, headaches, and other health issues."

How much is enough? A little over half, or about 55 percent, of your daily calories should come from carbohydrates, says Sass.

Eat more than that, especially from starchy carbs, and you risk changing your metabolism, adds Friel. "I test my athletes throughout the season, and when I see someone who has started eating lots of starch, they not only have gained fat, but they also have changed their metabolism from fat-burning to sugar-burning," he says. "It doesn't happen after one plate of pasta. But the body is very adaptable. Over the course of a couple of months, it will switch over to burn whatever you're feeding it most." The goal is to make (and keep) your body the most efficient fat burner it can be, so you burn more fat on every ride, store excess calories in easily accessible muscle stores, and can ride longer on less food without worrying about running out of energy.

WHERE THE CARBS ARE

VEGETABLES	CARBS (G)
Artichokes, cooked (1 medium)	13
Beets, cooked (½ cup)	8
Broccoli, raw (1 cup)	4
Brussels sprouts, cooked (½ cup)	7
Cabbage, cooked (½ cup)	3
Carrots, cooked (½ cup)	8
Cauliflower, cooked (½ cup)	3
Celery, raw (1 cup)	4
Chard, Swiss, cooked (1 cup)	7
Collard greens, cooked (1 cup)	12
Corn, sweet, cooked (1 oz)	7
Eggplant / aubergine, cooked (1 cup)	7
Kale, cooked (1 cup)	7
Leeks, cooked (½ cup)	4
Mushrooms, raw (1 cup)	4
Onions, raw (1 cup)	14
Parsnips, cooked (½ cup)	15
Peas, green, cooked (1 cup)	25
Peppers, green (1 cup)	10
Pumpkin, cooked, mashed (1 cup)	12
Radishes, raw (1 cup)	4
Spinach, cooked (1 cup)	7
Squash, winter, acorn, cooked (1 cup)	30

VEGETABLES (Contd.)	CARBS (G) (Contd.)
Squash, zucchini, cooked (1 cup)	8
Succotash, cooked (1 cup)	47
Sweet potato, baked w/ skin (1 large)	44
Tomatoes, raw (1 cup)	8
Turnip, cooked, mashed (1 cup)	11
FRUIT	**CARBS (G)**
Cantaloupe (1 cup)	15
Grapes (1 cup)	16
Honeydew (1 cup)	16
Kiwifruit (1 large)	14
Mangos (1 regular)	35
Nectarines (1 medium)	16
Oranges (1 medium)	14
Peaches (1 large)	17
Pears (1 medium)	25
Pineapple (1 cup)	19
Plums (1 medium)	8
Pomegranates, raw (1 medium)	26
Raisins, seedless (¼ cup)	32
Raspberries (1 cup)	14
Strawberries (1 cup)	11
Tangerines, mandarin oranges (1)	8
Watermelon (1 cup)	11
PASTA AND GRAINS	**CARBS (G)**
BREAD	
French (1 large slice)	18
Italian (1 large slice)	15
Mixed-grain (1 large slice)	15

(continued)

PASTA AND GRAINS (Contd.)	CARBS (G) (Contd.)
Pita, white (6" diameter)	33
Pita, whole wheat (6" diameter)	35
Pumpernickel (1 slice)	12
Rye (1 slice)	15
Sourdough (1 large slice)	18
Wheat (1 slice)	12
PASTA	
Macaroni (1 cup) cooked	40
Macaroni, whole wheat (1 cup) cooked	37
Spaghetti (1 cup) cooked	40
Spaghetti, whole wheat (1 cup) cooked	37
Tagliatelle (1 cup) cooked	44
RICE	
Long-grain brown (1 cup) cooked	45
Long-grain white (1 cup) cooked	45
Short-grain white (1 cup) cooked	37

When you do eat grains, pastas, cereals, and breads, be sure they're whole grains. A Pennsylvania State University study of overweight men and women found that those who ate a healthful diet that included whole grains, which are naturally higher in filling fiber than their refined counterparts, lost significantly more health-wrecking abdominal fat after 12 weeks than those who ate refined grains.

Finally, pair those carbs with protein whenever possible. Lean meats, nut butters, fish, and eggs slow down digestion so you feel full sooner, get more even energy from your meals, and stay full longer. The amino acids in protein also help repair, build, and maintain muscle tissue.

✳PICK UP THE PROTEIN

Traditionally, cyclists haven't placed as high of a premium on protein as power sport athletes, like sprinters and football players, have. But for both performance and weight-loss purposes, protein is a key player in the *Ride Your Way Lean* diet.

"There are far too many endurance athletes who emphasize carbs to the exclusion of all else, which frankly can lead to all kinds of weight and performance issues," says Bonci. (While most of us know that protein is important for building and repairing muscle, we don't realize that it also helps build immunity; protects essential tissues during endurance activity like long, hard rides; blunts your appetite; and even helps you burn more calories just by eating it.)

Protein is composed of 20 different amino acids, all of which act as the building blocks for your muscles. During long rides, hard interval efforts, and resistance training, your muscles take a bit of a beating. That's a good thing provided that you feed them enough amino acids to repair and come back stronger, which, of course, is where protein comes in. Adding protein to your diet can help reduce the damage and ease the aches. Though it's not a primary fuel source, protein does supply some much-needed energy for your churning pistons, especially as your glycogen supplies run low, says Bonci. "During endurance exercise, 3 to 8 percent of energy needs are supplied by branched-chain amino acids [BCAAs], specifically leucine, isoleucine, and valine, that are found in many protein-rich foods," she says. "These are the BCAAs that skeletal muscle oxidizes for energy." Without adequate amounts your performance suffers, and your ride feels harder.

In one study published in the *European Journal of Applied Physiology*, researchers found that canoeists who took leucine supplements for 6 weeks improved the time they could row until exhaustion by a whopping 11 minutes, while they also lowered their rate of perceived exertion (RPE), how hard they felt they were working, by nearly two points, from "hard" to "somewhat hard." A similar group of rowers who took dummy pills over the same time frame enjoyed no such performance benefits. What's more: Research suggests that BCAAs also may boost immunity, lift mood, and sharpen mental function during endurance activities, like long bike rides.

On the weight-loss front, research shows that protein improves satiety and revs up your metabolism because it takes more work for your body to digest and process. While carbs generally increase your metabolism by 5 to 15 percent after you eat them, protein sends it soaring 20 to 35 percent. Leucine, in particular, seems to help athletes keep precious muscle tissue as they shed fat. A study reported in the *Journal of Nutrition* found that substituting some high-quality protein foods like meats, dairy, eggs, and nuts for high-carb fare such as breads, pasta, and potatoes accelerated fat loss and helped maintain lean muscle tissue in exercisers who were trying to drop pounds.

FOOD	PROTEIN (G)
BUTTER	
Almond (2 Tbsp)	4
Cashew (2 Tbsp)	6
Peanut (2 Tbsp)	8
OTHER DAIRY PRODUCTS	
Cheese (2 oz)	14
Eggs (2)	7
Low-fat milk (1 cup)	8
MEATS	
Beef (3 oz)	21
Chicken breast (4 oz)	35
Pork chop (3 oz)	24
Turkey (3 oz)	25

FOOD	PROTEIN (G)
FISH AND SHELLFISH	
Salmon (3 oz)	19
Shrimp (3 oz)	18
Tuna (6-oz can)	40
Whitefish (3 oz)	16
SOY PRODUCTS	
Lentils (1 cup, cooked)	18
Soy milk (1 cup)	11
Tofu, firm (½ block)	26

Endurance athletes should eat a minimum of 0.5 gram of protein for every pound of body weight, which is easy to remember, since the number is just half your body weight. The average American often comes in a little shy of that amount; don't let yourself be one of them. Sports nutrition experts also recommend eating about 20 grams of BCAAs every day. Again, it's completely unrealistic to think you'll be scouring labels and tallying up BCAA grams. The easier thing to do is to include protein-rich foods with every meal. Most of the time, especially on the days when you're not riding, focus meals on vegetables, fruits, and lean proteins. One caveat is to avoid high-fat foods masquerading as protein, such as fast-food burgers and highly processed meats. Super sources include lean meat, poultry, fish, soy foods, dairy, and nuts. Vegetarians can substitute beans and rice (1 cup of each contains about 20 grams of protein) and soy foods for animal products.

✳MAKE YOUR FAT A MUFA

It's no coincidence that the collective weight of the nation has gone up with the growing popularity of low-fat and "lite" foods. "For decades the government was preaching that we should get as much fat as possible out of our diet and replace it with carbohydrates. This wasn't only misguided. It was flat out wrong, especially for athletes," says Friel. "As your body becomes more conditioned, you become a better fat burner. You need ample amounts of healthy fat, which contrary to popular belief, won't make you fat. Starchy foods turn to fat far easier."

What's more, evidence is mounting that eating plenty of healthy unsaturated fats is essential for firing up your fat-burning metabolism. Most recently, Harvard researchers studied 101 women, putting half of them on a low-fat diet and half on a diet that included about 20 percent of calories from monounsaturated fatty acids (MUFAs). After 18 months, the MUFA-eating group dropped 11 pounds, compared to their low-fat-eating peers, who shed only 6 pounds. Fat is also slower to digest than carbs, so it helps you stay hunger free longer. Eating a healthy dose of fat may also help you ride longer, so you can burn more calories and lose more weight, says Friel. Research shows that athletes who eat about a third of their daily calories from healthy fats are able to keep cranking longer before getting exhausted in exercise tests than those who eat a low-fat, high-carb diet.

MUFAs may also help you be healthier and live longer. Research shows they can help prevent and control type 2 diabetes, lower your risk of heart disease, and help reduce inflammation in the body, which lowers your risk for a host of diseases as well as speeds exercise recovery. Sass recommends getting about 20 percent of your calories from MUFAs, or about 50 grams a day if you're eating 2,000 calories a day. Don't worry about getting too hung up on counting calorie percentages and fat grams, however. A simple way to make sure you get enough MUFAs in your diet is to include one MUFA-rich food, like almonds, avocado, and olive oil, at every meal. The best strategy is to replace some of your refined carbs with a MUFA-rich food. Try nuts and seeds, olive spreads like tapenade, avocado, and the occasional chunk of dark chocolate. Some healthy portions to shoot for:

- **Nuts and seeds:** Try mixed nuts, seeds, and nut butters like almond, cashew, and tahini. A serving size is 2 tablespoons.

- **Olives:** Black, green, mixed, or blended in a spreadable tapenade. A serving is 10 large olives or 2 tablespoons of tapenade.

- **Oils:** Canola, flaxseed, peanut, safflower, walnut, sunflower, sesame, or olive. Cook with them; drizzle them; eat them in pesto. One serving is 1 tablespoon.

- **Avocado:** Serve as guacamole or just slice and eat. One-quarter cup equals one serving.

- **Dark chocolate:** Must be dark or semisweet. Aim for $\frac{1}{4}$ cup or about 2 ounces.

Other healthy fat sources include those rich in omega-3 fatty acids, like fatty fish. Originally called "vitamin F," omega-3 fatty acids are part of a family called polyunsaturated fatty acids (PUFAs, the sister fat to MUFAs). PUFAs come in two forms, omega-6 and omega-3. Your body can't make or store either, so you have to eat them regularly. Omega-6s are no problem for most of us; in fact, we go overboard with them, since they're found in vegetable oils like corn, sunflower, safflower, cottonseed, and soybean, which are plentiful in snack foods, fast foods, and processed foods including cereal, soups, and more. Omega-3s are far more difficult to come by. They're found in nuts (which also contain omega-6 acids) and some plants. The single best source, however, is fish. And the last time you ate fish was when?

"Unless you're making a concentrated effort, and that means eating fish several times a week, you are just not getting enough omega-3s," says Bonci. Omega-3s may be even more important for active people because they help reduce inflammation in the body, which means faster recovery and overall better health, she says. "I see clients who take anti-inflammatory meds like ibuprofen every day. They shouldn't. Instead, they should try having enough omega-3s on board to help head off the inflammatory process and potentially prevent delayed onset muscle soreness and joint inflammation, not to mention improve general health." How much is enough? About 1,000 to 2,000 milligrams a day. See the amount in these common foods to determine how your omega-3 intake is stacking up. If it's not so hot, add some of these to your weekly diet, and aim to eat fish at least two or three times a week.

FOOD	OMEGA-3 (MG)
Anchovies (3 oz)	1,750
Eggs (omega-3-fortified, 2)	114
Lean beef (3 oz, grass-fed)	136
Mackerel (3 oz)	1,120
Salmon (3 oz)	1,830
Tuna (3 oz)	1,280

You'll note I didn't talk too much about "bad fats." That's because what defines a bad fat is constantly changing. Not that long ago doctors were pretty much telling us all fat was bad. That, as we now know, was a big fat mistake. Saturated fat wore the devil's horns for many years. But new research shows that though saturated fats may be less healthy as a whole, they're not all bad. In fact, some of them may be good for you. Coconut oil, which is a saturated fat, appears to behave more like an unsaturated fat in the body. Certain saturated fats found in lean meats may even help improve your cholesterol, rather than raise it as previously thought. The best advice is to follow the recommendations for healthy fats above, which include foods that naturally contain some not-so-bad-for-you saturated fats.

The one fat everyone agrees you should avoid is trans fat. Entire cities, if not states, are passing legislation to ban them, so you know they're probably pretty bad. The biggest trouble with them is they're almost entirely unnatural. They are vegetable oils that are highly processed with hydrogen gas to solidify them (hence the name on the label: hydrogenated or partially hydrogenated vegetable oil). They're so foreign to anything found in nature that our bodies literally don't know how to process them, and we end up wearing them around the insides of our arteries and, according to a growing body of literature, around our waistlines. Research suggests that trans fats promote weight gain and encourage the body to store more dangerous abdominal fat, even if you're not overeating calories. Up until recently, these fabricated fat disasters were found in practically every processed food on the shelves, including crackers, cookies, cakes, chips, margarines, and more. But food manufacturers have been making concerted efforts to eliminate them.

MAXIMIZE YOUR MICRONUTRIENTS

If macronutrients like carbs, fat, and protein are your body's fuel, micronutrients like vitamins and minerals are the ignition wires and spark plugs that transform that fuel into high-octane energy and transport it to all the places it needs to go to power you down the road. As an active cyclist, you need to get at least the recommended Daily Value for all your vitamins and minerals, but there are a few that deserve extra attention.

B vitamins. Sports nutrition studies show that active people don't perform their best and have trouble building muscle and producing oxygen-carrying red blood cells when they're low in B vitamins like B_6, B_{12}, folate, and riboflavin, which are essential for converting protein and sugar to energy and for repairing cells. You burn through your B vitamins when you're on long rides and when you're exercising lots, so be sure to fill up on vitamin B–dense foods such as dark green leafy veggies, fish and shellfish, legumes, whole grains, and low-fat dairy.

Iron. Iron is essential for forming red blood cells, which in turn carry oxygen to your working muscles. Without enough of this blood-building mineral, you succumb to anemia, a fatigue-causing condition that will leave you too pooped to pedal, strength-train, or do any real calorie-burning activity of any kind. Women are especially vulnerable to low iron levels. In fact, a study from Italy found that active women have lower iron stores than their couch potato peers. Fortify yourself with seafood, fish, lean meat, poultry, nuts, fortified grains, beans and lentils, and dark green leafy vegetables.

Calcium. The average adult gets only about 700 milligrams of calcium a day, well shy of the recommended 800 milligrams to 1,200 milligrams needed. As a cyclist, you may need even more since your body doesn't just use calcium to build bone, it also relies on a steady supply of this electrolyte mineral to keep your muscles firing smoothly, regulate your blood pressure, and maintain healthy nerve function. If you don't feed your body all the calcium it needs, it goes mining for it from your bones—bad news if you want to maintain a strong skeleton. Eat three servings of low-fat dairy foods like yogurt, fat-free milk, and low-fat cheese every day.

Consuming a little more dairy each day may also help you shed more fat. Dairy foods help you feel fuller, so you're less likely to overeat, says Cindy Dallow, PhD, RD, who operates Partners in Nutrition, a nutritional consulting firm in Loveland, Colorado. Research also shows that consuming the recommended dose of calcium each day cranks up your fat-burning metabolism to high. In one study, dieters who ate a high-dairy diet (1,200 to 1,300 milligrams a day) lost nearly twice as much weight as their non-dairy-eating peers on a 24-week weight-loss program.

Antioxidants. Much has been made of antioxidants, such as vitamins C and E and beta-carotene, over the past couple of decades. We know they fight free radicals—cell-damaging molecules that have been linked to cancer, heart disease, and other chronic illnesses. They neutralize the free radicals we create during hard exercise and help reduce muscle damage. There's no question they're essential for good health. But it remains pretty questionable whether or not taking them in supplement form is helpful,or perhaps even harmful. Scientists had to pull the plug on early beta-carotene studies because they found that smokers popping these pills were actually increasing their risk for cancer. It's not that beta-carotene is harmful; it's that antioxidants work together in ways we still don't understand, so taking megadoses of one at the expense of others may not be such a great idea, according to current literature. Your best bet? You guessed it. Food, especially fruits and vegetables, in its pure form, which naturally contains antioxidants in all the right disease-fighting blends.

In case you haven't noticed the trend, the easiest way to get all the essential nutrients you need is to eat whole, natural, recognizable foods and lots of them. Coach James Herrera puts it simply: Do not focus on specific macronutrient balance (protein, carbs, fat). Rather, focus on eating the most nutrient-dense, unprocessed foods you can. He says your primary food categories should be vegetables (leafy greens such as spinach, cabbage, bok choy, and arugula are incredibly high in nutrient density), fruits, legumes, nuts, seeds, whole grains, and modest amounts of animal protein, with a focus on organic, grass fed, and free range when possible.

Here are Coach Herrara's top five foods for filling up on all the micronutrients you need. You can't go wrong with any of these.

Vegetables. Eat leafy greens daily. A great way to do this is to put together a huge salad as a meal. Start with a base of leafy greens, then include a variety of shapes and colors like carrots, tomatoes, mushrooms, peppers, olives, legumes, fruit (if you're so inclined), nuts, and seeds. Throughout the day, try to include vegetables in your diet as snacks (baby carrots, snap peas, grape tomatoes, and cut-up peppers are great) and as a major component to entrées. Another thing you need to focus on here is letting the vegetables comprise the largest area on your plate. For example, when making something like spaghetti, use half the pasta (whole grain, of course), but make the sauce rich with as many vegetables as you'd like. You'll still fill your belly, but you'll also enjoy the benefits of all those extra vitamins, minerals, antioxidants, and phytosterols from your veggies.

Fruits. Don't skimp here or adhere to the measly 2 cups a day recommended by the food pyramid. Buy lots of fresh fruit, keep it washed and readily available, then enjoy as much as you'd like daily. Shoot for four to six pieces of fruit, each from a different family and/or color. If your favorite fresh fruits aren't in season, look for the frozen variety with no added sugar or syrup—smoothie time.

Legumes. A great source of protein, legumes like peas, beans, lentils, and peanuts are high in fiber and very filling. Everyone knows black beans and chickpeas, but dig in and really experiment with the bean family. You'll find a wide array of flavors and textures from pinto, kidney, soy, adzuki, navy, green, northern, white, and lima beans. A multibean soup or chili is a great way to add legumes to your diet. Snack on roasted, unsalted soybeans; put beans in a tortilla wrap with avocado, spinach, and tomato; or add kidney beans and chickpeas to a salad.

Nuts. These perfect snack packages contain an abundance of protein and omega-3 fatty acids. Enjoy a wide variety of nuts, such as almonds, Brazil nuts, cashews, chestnuts, walnuts, pecans, and pine nuts, but remember, they're still high in calories. It's easy to get a large number of calories in a handful. Space out your intake throughout the day, or use them as an added topping to steel-cut oats, muesli, whole-grain-flour pancakes, and salads, or as a daytime snack.

Seeds. Often overlooked and underappreciated, seeds like pumpkin and sunflower seeds are nutritional powerhouses packed with essential micronutrients, especially minerals. Flaxseed is also rich in omega-3 fatty acids. Add some to your cereal, salads, smoothies, and other dishes.

DRINK UP

About 60 percent of you is made up of water. Only 10 percent of that water is coursing through your veins as part of your bloodstream. That may not seem like important information until you consider that you can easily lose 1 to 2 percent of your water weight during a warm summer ride. Because pedaling through the air whisks the sweat off your skin so quickly, it's also easy not to register the fluid loss, until it's too late.

Even slight dehydration can cause performance to plummet, as water is lost from the bloodstream. As your blood volume decreases, your heart has to work harder. Research shows that for every pound of sweat you lose, your heart rate increases about eight beats per minute. You also run the risk of becoming overheated, as your body's ability to sweat and cool itself diminishes. Heavier riders are particularly vulnerable since they tend to sweat more and are already at risk for overheating and overexertion. There's also good evidence that less-conditioned people, like those just starting out in cycling, may be more sensitive to the potentially detrimental effects of dehydration than their more-conditioned counterparts. Finally, staying hydrated is a must when you're trying to lose weight because water helps your body metabolize fat.

How much fluid is enough? You'll find answers all over the map. As a general rule, experts say you should drink about $1^1/_2$ to 2 quarts of fluid a day, more when you're going to be out riding long and/or hard in the heat (see "Eat to Ride" for more specific guidelines on how much and what to drink during cycling). Though water is ideal, the notion that you must drink 8 cups of water a day has pretty much been filed under "urban legend." No one really knows where the idea came from, and experts generally agree there's no scientific foundation for it. In fact, you can get your fluids in many forms, including juices, soups, teas, and even coffee (though, sorry, not alcohol). That's right. Contrary to what you may have heard about the dehydrating effects of caffeine, that's simply not true. Yes, if you have 30 ounces of coffee in the morning, you're going to pee more. But that would also be true of the same amount of orange juice or any fluid. That's great news for cyclists because, as you'll soon learn, caffeine can give you a real performance boost on the bike.

You may even consider getting some of your H_2O quota by piling your plate with more water-rich foods like tomatoes, lettuce, oranges, melons, cucumbers, peaches, and plums. Research suggests that the more water-rich foods you eat, the easier it is to lose weight. In one Japanese study, simply drinking more water didn't help a group of women lose weight, but eating more juicy foods did, perhaps because these foods also contain fiber (but not many calories), so you're more likely to feel full faster and eat less overall.

One thing you should avoid in the hydration equation is too many empty calories from sodas, sweetened drinks like packaged ice tea, and alcohol. Try to substitute less sugary, more nutritious alternatives like juice with no added sugar, milk, or fizzy waters for these beverages. Avoid making the common mistake of simply drinking diet versions of these drinks instead. Research shows that artificial sweeteners may prove even worse for your waistline because, like processed fats, your body doesn't know what to do with them. In an 8-year study of more than 1,500 men and women ages 25 to 64, University of Texas researchers found that for each diet soft drink they drank, their risk for becoming overweight rose 41 percent. The study researchers speculate that artificial sweeteners may prime your tastebuds, and maybe even your brain, to crave the real thing—sugary treats, which could unconsciously cause you to eat more sweets or high-carb foods than you otherwise would.

EAT TO RIDE

Cycling is a killer calorie burner. But if you're not careful, you can still easily eat more than you use up. "Cyclists notoriously overestimate their calorie burn," says Bonci. "It's important to be careful with your pre-, during, and post-ride nutrition, especially if you're trying to lose weight, because if you eat an energy bar and drink a sports drink on a moderate ride, you have effectively cancelled out any calories you burned."

In general, if you're just going for an easy to moderate hour-long ride, you don't need any special fuel. Just plan your day's snack so it's within an hour of your ride and enjoy the spin, eating as usual for the rest of the day. When you're going to be riding longer and/or harder, as well as including strength-training, you'll want to fuel properly not just so you'll perform optimally but also so you don't end up ravenous at the end of the day, eating everything within arm's reach.

Nearly all experts agree, one of the easiest ways to avoid overeating, especially when you're ramping up your activity to lose weight, is to time your eating so you give your body fuel when it needs it. Think of it like gassing up your car. You don't start out close to E, drive it until it's empty, then push it to the nearest Mobil and pump gas into it until it's overflowing and trickling down the tarmac. You make sure the tank is adequately filled before you pull out, then top it off as needed along the way, maybe putting a little back in at the end of the trip so it's ready to roll the next morning. The following guidelines will help you eat just right for the energy you need without the excess calories you don't.

Front-Load Your Fueling

As mentioned above, you want to stock your muscle stores before you ride rather than start out low and play catch-up the rest of the day (which inevitably ends up in overeating). Of course, you also don't want a full meal sitting like a lump in your gut when you're trying to pedal fast. So the trick is to give yourself just enough time to digest, but not so much that your liver glycogen and blood sugar levels start to drop and you're ready for your next meal. My magic number for pre-ride eating is 3 hours. That gives you time to eat a good meal, yet still be comfortably digested when it's time to saddle up. For small- to medium-size meals or snacks, you can safely eat 90 minutes to 2 hours before rolling.

What you eat is just as important as when. Now is the time to treat yourself to some carbohydrates (though not exactly license to drive through Dunkin' Donuts). If you're going to ride longer than 90 minutes, you can double the carbohydrates you'd usually eat. Ideally you want to shoot for 40 to 100 grams of carbohydrates in the hours before a long ride. A peanut butter and honey sandwich is a great example of a healthy, high-carb, and nutrient-dense pre-ride meal. Though a little fat and protein is ok, foods that are very high in either of these can cause a holdup in your digestive system and slow your stomach emptying.

By eating before you ride, you'll also burn more calories during your ride. Sports science researchers have found that exercise burns more calories after a meal than it does during a fasting state, which makes perfect sense if you think about how the body is designed to protect itself during periods of famine. When you're well-fueled, you simply have more energy, so you're able to put more power into your pedals and get more out of your ride than if you go into it flagging from low-blood-sugar fatigue. A few ideal pre-ride snacks or minimeals:

• Banana with yogurt

• Cereal and milk

• Crackers and peanut butter

• Energy bar (i.e., Clif or PowerBar with about 250 calories)

• Fig bars and milk

• Oatmeal and raisins

Top Off as You Go

For any rides longer than 90 minutes to 2 hours, pack a snack. After that point, you'll have burned through your glycogen stores and will start to feel like you're running on fumes. Now is when simple sugars are A-OK because they're easy to digest and will shoot into your bloodstream quickly, providing instant energy to keep pedaling. Remember, your brain runs on glycogen. It will say unhappy things to you (like "Quit now!") if you don't feed it during a long ride.

How much is enough? Studies show that 30 to 60 grams of carbs (or about 120 to 240 calories) an hour significantly boosts endurance performance. One energy gel like GU or half an energy bar (see "Drinks, Bars, and Gels," on page 118) provides about 30 grams of carbs and 120 calories. Wash it down with some energy drink, which delivers about 14 grams of carbs and 50 calories in 8 ounces, and you're good to keep going. Sports drinks also have the advantage of helping to keep you hydrated, so you get a two-for-one benefit by putting one in your bottle. What's more, researchers have found that exercisers who keep their blood sugar levels high by sipping a sports drink feel happier and more energized than those who plow forward on plain water alone.

That said, though bars and gels and drinks are convenient ways to meet your on-the-go carb needs, don't think that you need to go out and buy special snacks and drinks. You can easily meet your needs with real food and water and ride just as happily, if not even more so, because real food often tastes better and costs less to boot. A few perfect portable snacks include a banana, fig bars, oatmeal cookies (I once did a 6-hour race on nothing but), peanut butter crackers, and peanut butter and jelly.

When Recovery Counts

Again, if you've just been out for a casual hour or two, you really don't have to worry about special recovery foods, especially if you also were fueling along the ride. If you were riding longer or doing intervals, however, you need to restock your glycogen stores so your muscles can recover and repair (and so you don't end up eating everything in arm's reach come your next meal).

The best time to replenish your muscle stores is within 2 hours, but ide-ally within 30 minutes, of finishing your ride because that's when your enzymes are most active and can most effectively shuttle the food you eat where it needs to go. This quick refueling strategy will also help you lose weight faster. For one, your body is working to put the calories you eat back into your muscles and liver rather than storing them as fat. In fact, your body burns more fat when you eat after exercise, so it can spare the carbo-hydrates that it is trying to replenish. What's more, your metabolism is still elevated from the exercise bout, so you're burning more calories overall during this time.

You can buy special recovery bars and drinks, but it's unnecessary for most recreational riders. What your body needs is carbohydrates for glycogen, protein for repair, and fluid for rehydration. All of those are easily obtained through fresh, real food. If you've finished a ride close to a meal, simply recover with that meal, being sure to emphasize healthy carbs and protein. If you're hours away from lunch or dinner, have a simple snack, similar to what you might eat before a ride. A glass of chocolate milk often can do the trick. Or, go with one of Herrera's favorite recovery foods and make a smoothie.

"Smoothies are one of the best ways to increase your fruit consumption, and they're hydrating, refreshing, and easy to make," he says. In a good blender, throw in crushed ice, a variety of berries (blackberries, blueberries, raspberries, strawberries, etc.), pineapple, banana, orange, pomegranate, whatever you have on hand. If your favorite fresh fruits aren't in season, look for the frozen variety with no added sugar or syrup. To help liquefy the mixture, use a bit of 100% fruit juice. For added omega-3s, throw in a tablespoon of ground flaxseed. Mix in a little nut butter, yogurt, or soy milk for some protein. Blend it all together and you're good to go. Since mixing up all those ingredients and cleaning the blender can be a bit of a hassle to do every day, blend enough to make two or three servings, then chill the extra in the refrigerator to enjoy the next day.

Bring a Bottle . . . or Two

Most bikes come with attachments for at least one, usually two, water bottles. Use them. Remember, hydration is important not just for on-the-bike performance but also for weight loss, so you want to keep the fluids flowing. A general rule of thumb is you should be draining about one 12- to 16-ounce water bottle every hour—that means drinking 3 to 4 ounces (or mouthfuls) every 15 to 20 minutes. You'll want even more fluid when riding in very hot conditions. The goal is not to replace every ounce of fluid you sweat out—that's impossible—but to stay ahead of dehydration.

For short rides, especially in moderate temperatures, plain water is fine. For anything longer than an hour, or even an hour-long ride in the heat of summer, bring a sports drink. Every pound of sweat you lose takes with it a host of essential electrolytes like sodium, potassium, calcium, and magnesium, which work in concert to keep your muscles firing smoothly, regulate nerve transmission, and maintain your body's fluid balance. When your electrolyte levels dip too low, you can suffer cramping, nausea, and fatigue. Sports drinks are specially formulated to replace the electrolytes you lose as well as refuel your muscles with carbohydrates. They also hydrate better than plain water because they contain sodium, which encourages you to drink more and helps your body retain the fluids that it takes in.

Jive with Java

You'll notice that bike rides often start at, finish at, and sometimes take breaks at coffee shops. There's a good reason for that. Caffeine is a natural turbocharger for cycling performance. The amount from just 2 cups of java frees up fatty acids to deliver easy-to-access energy in your bloodstream as well as boosts your body's ability to burn fat and spare carbohydrates during long rides. This popular pick-me-up also helps you push harder with less pain. A British review of 21 caffeine studies revealed that caffeinated exercisers not only reported lower ratings of perceived exertion (RPE—how hard exercise feels) but also were able to run, swim, bike, and row 11 percent faster and/or longer before tiring out.

If you don't drink coffee or you're sensitive to caffeine, don't feel the need to start just for a performance benefit. But if you're a regular joe drinker, you can feel good about using your daily fix to your advantage. Sports nutritionist studies show that drinking about 3 to 6 milligrams per kilogram (1 kilogram = 2.2 pounds) of body weight 1 hour before you ride can improve your endurance. In plain English that's a 10-ounce cup of coffee for a 150-pound rider. Or even more simply put, just toss back about 200 to 300 milligrams (a double or triple espresso or about 16 ounces of brewed coffee) 1 hour before go time.

❋SECRETS OF THE SLIM CYCLISTS

Look around a group of enviably thin cyclists, and you might assume they're naturally lean or that it comes easily. But rest assured, most riders, like most people, have had their share of ups and downs on the scale. You might imagine that as a certified coach, trainer, athlete, and *Bicycling's* "Fit Chick," I'd have figured out the weight thing long ago. But as I confessed in the Introduction, until fairly recently, the numbers on the scale would bounce around like a faulty shock and, despite doing "everything right," I would often find myself stuck with 5 to 10 pounds that weren't contributing to the useful portion of the power-to-weight equation.

My main problem was that, like millions of cyclists, I was a high-carb consumer. To me, if it didn't end with an "i" (rotini, tortellini, fusilli), it wasn't fuel. I had never stopped to think that carbs come in many shapes and sizes, or that as a cyclist, I actually burned a lot of fat for fuel. Then I started doing some searching around and read many of the philosophies and principles regarding carbs that I've outlined in this chapter. I read with great interest about how Allen Lim, PhD, of Team Radio Shack and the brains behind much of Garmin-Slipstream's training and race preparation had eliminated wheat from the Tour riders' diets and was feeding them rice cakes topped with eggs, olive oil, prosciutto, and liquid amino acids. I talked with Joe Friel, the king of advocating carbohydrates in his TrainingBible series, about his own complete 180-degree turn away from starches and move toward vegetables, fruits, and lean meats as fuel so that he would become a better fat, instead of sugar, burner. I started to understand why I hit the wall so often out of the blue, bonked on my bike, and was hungry again 30 minutes post morning bagel.

With nothing to lose but those nagging 10 pounds, I overhauled my eating. Good-bye, "-ini" foods (except for side dishes before a big ride or the night before a race). Hello, broccoli, Brussels sprouts, leafy greens, nuts, fruit, and lean meats. Within a couple of months I went from the mid-130s to the mid-120s. And there I have stayed, nearly effortlessly. The best part: I rarely even come close to bonking, and I feel like I can ride much longer on far less food. Which got me wondering what other secrets cyclists can use to successfully (and nearly effortlessly) maintain their weight. Here's a roundup from nutritionists, researchers, and coaches.

Get It Right in the Grocery Store

You can't find yourself scraping the crumbs off the bottom of a bag of chips unless you buy that bag of chips. Sounds simple. But it's a mistake most of us make. We bring foods into the house that will do nothing but sabotage our weight-loss efforts. After one too many empty jar episodes, I learned that Nutella is something that can't be in my pantry. I simply find it irresistible. I may buy some other treat that is more manageable, but I make a concerted effort to fill my cart with foods that will make me feel good and that I'll feel good about eating. Getting it right at the grocery store is something James Herrera emphasizes as the first most important step toward eating right and losing weight.

"When you're hungry, you go to the kitchen and look in the refrigerator and pantry and grab whatever is there," he says. "If it's accessible, you're going to eat it. If healthy food choices are readily available, you're far less likely to make a bad choice." Do yourself a favor and just don't buy nutritionally barren food that you know you can't resist after a long day at the office or while chilling with your favorite TV shows. Create an environment where it's easy to succeed. Create a fruit bowl. Buy prechopped veggies and hummus and keep them in the refrigerator at all times. Stock your pantry with nuts and seeds.

Likewise, keep healthy snacks readily available at all times. "If you have a bag of mixed nuts or a banana in your bag, you're far less likely to be tempted by the drive-thru when you get hungry on your way home," says Herrera. Keep snacks in easily accessible places, like your desk drawer, your glove compartment, your purse, or your work bag, so they're there in case of a hunger emergency. Good choices are small energy bars like Lärabars and dried fruit and nut mixes.

Put Down the Packages

Many people—even otherwise active people—think they're eating healthfully, when in reality they consume far more sugar, sodium, preservatives, additives, and maybe even trans fats than they realize because they eat so many packaged crackers, cereals, snack bars, and other processed foods. Added sugar is particularly problematic if you're trying to lose weight because it causes your body to step up its production of insulin, which in turn blocks hormones that control appetite. As a result, the food you eat is quickly stored as fat and you're always hungry.

Unfortunately, you can't even choose wisely by reading the box. In a *New York Times* essay, food writer Michael Pollan laments that Froot Loops have earned a Smart Choices check mark from the FDA, branding it a cereal that is a good choice for healthy eating. To which he (and I and most other reasoned folks) say, "Really?" Don't buy it. The major food manufacturers have far too much pull in food labeling and marketing and, yes, even government recommendations. It's far better to trust your instincts: If it doesn't look like real food, it's probably not the healthiest choice.

Eat mostly whole foods that you recognize as part of an animal or plant, says sports nutritionist and exercise physiologist Tavis Piattoly, RD, LD, assistant general manager at Elmwood Fitness Center in New Orleans. "The vast majority of foods in the grocery store are processed, packaged junk," he says. For the healthiest grocery store fare, shop around the perimeter of the store first. That's where they stock the fresh produce, meats, poultry, fish, dairy, grains, and other whole foods. By the time you reach the interior aisles, where all the packaged foods are, your cart should be pretty full. Top it off with healthy packaged foods like nuts, tuna fish, fresh sauces, spices, frozen fruit and vegetables, and other makings for healthful meals.

Eat (a Lot) Early

It's repeated more often than *It's a Wonderful Life* at Christmastime, but somehow the message still isn't getting through. According to a survey by the International Food Information Council Foundation, fewer than half of us eat a morning meal daily. That's a big mistake. During the night, you've gone 8, maybe more, hours without food, yet your body is still humming along, repairing muscle tissue, fighting disease, dreaming dreams while you sleep. By the time you awaken, your glycogen stores are low. You need to eat something to fire up your metabolism, or your body will be running on fumes. Worse, you'll go into an energy deficit that not only leaves you ravenous (and more likely to overeat) later on but also suppresses your calorie-burning furnaces, so you're more likely to send all those calories you throw down straight into storage. It's simply your body's way of protecting itself from what it perceives as potential starvation.

Research shows that people who blow off breakfast are $4^1/_2$ times more likely to be overweight than those who faithfully eat a morning meal. "It's one of the biggest fueling mistakes everyone, including athletes, makes," says Piattoly. "Most athletes overeat at dinner and through the evening because they don't eat enough earlier in the day to fuel their efforts. The result: Your hunger steadily increases as your energy levels decrease, and you end up overeating and sending fuel into fat storage instead of burning it on your bike."

The solution is to eat more in the morning. Since you have a whole day of activity and, on most days, a good ride ahead of you, try to eat about 25 percent of your daily calories in the morning hours. Breakfast should include protein, healthy fat, and fiber-rich carbs like fruit. A British study found that exercisers who ate a fiber-rich breakfast burned twice as much fat during subsequent workouts later in the day than those who ate more refined (less fibrous) foods. "Refined carbohydrates spike your insulin levels, which makes it harder for your body to use fat as fuel," says Lisa Dorfman, RD, CSSD, sports nutritionist, and adjunct professor at the University of Miami.

For a power breakfast that'll sustain you well into the day, try two eggs, any style, $^1/_2$ cup whole oats (cooked), 1 cup yogurt, and 1 cup mixed berries with coffee and OJ. In fact, eggs may be a key to long-term weight loss.

When researchers from Louisiana State University's Pennington Biomedical Research Center fed 160 overweight men and women a 340-calorie breakfast of eggs and toast or a 340-calorie bagel breakfast 5 days a week for 8 weeks, those who started the day with protein-packed eggs lost about twice as much weight as those who breakfasted on bagels. What's more, egg breakfast dieters shrank their waistlines 83 percent more than their carb-only counterparts. Other studies have found that egg eaters consume fewer calories all day long than those starting the day with other breakfast foods. "Eggs are a great source of protein and good fat, as well as iron and other important nutrients," says Bonci. "When you start the day with them, you're more likely to eat less all day."

Eat Often

People skip meals thinking it's an easy way to cut back on calories. But it almost always backfires. Skipping meals encourages bingeing and crushes your willpower. Try to eat every 3 to 4 hours, and never go more than 4 to 5 hours without food, recommends Piattoly. It helps you control your hunger and manage your appetite.

Most diets treat hunger like the enemy. But it's your closest ally in the battle of the bulge, says Piattoly. "Once you start the fat reduction process, you're going to be a little hungry, but not starving," he says. "The trick is learning to balance the two, so you're losing weight but not setting yourself up for a binge. Eat breakfast, then wait until you feel hungry and eat just until you're no longer hungry," he says. "That's where people usually go wrong. They eat way past the point of satisfaction until they're 'full.' Eat only until you're no longer hungry. Then wait 3 to 4 hours and you should feel hungry again. If not, you ate too much earlier. If you're starving in an hour, you didn't eat enough," he explains. It takes a while to get the hang of it, but once you do, weight loss and ultimately maintenance is much easier.

"After trying many different diets and weight-loss programs, I discovered the key to lasting weight loss was that it had to be fun—riding a bike—and sustainable, which means not starving yourself," says Mark Blaubach, 41, who at 31 years of age found himself at a very unhappy 364 pounds. "I found the best way to abate extreme hunger and subsequent bingeing was to never let my blood sugar fall enough to make me really hungry," says Mark, who has kept off more than 100 pounds. "For me that meant definitely not going too long without food. I would eat a small, balanced high-protein meal every 3 to 4 hours."

This strategy also means planning your snacks instead of just letting them happen when hunger hits. By planning to have some yogurt and trail mix at 10:30 a.m. and a chunk of dark chocolate at 3 p.m., you also free your head from thinking about food. When you feel a little hungry, you can calm your brain with the assurance that there's a balanced meal or a satisfying snack right around the corner. Likewise, don't be afraid to have a little bed-time snack if you find yourself ravenous at night. A small snack like a little oatmeal not only will generate some feel-good brain chemicals that will help you relax and fall asleep but also will keep you from waking up hungry (so you get more quality sleep) and potentially raiding the fridge.

EMOTIONAL EATING

It would be naïve at best and ignorant at worst to presume that all you need is knowledge to eat a healthy, balanced diet. Let's face it, we all know that plowing through a bag of sour cream and onion potato chips is going to put a dent in our weight-loss efforts, but we do it anyway. Why we find our hand scraping crumbs from the bottom of a once-full bag has nothing to do with being hungry or not knowing that carrots and hummus would be a more slimming snack choice. We do it because those chips feed something in our brain, not our belly. They make us feel happy. Or at least dampen what is making us feel sad, frustrated, angry, or (insert negative emotion of your choice here). They also help us celebrate when we're feeling happy. Many of us wash down nearly every emotion with a heaping serving of our favorite foods.

You can't do much to control your feelings (though riding your bike more should certainly help lift your spirits). But you can control how you respond to them, says Sass. "Eating feels good in the moment and can be one of the easiest, most accessible ways to cope with your feelings," she acknowledges. But that type of coping isn't conducive to losing weight. The key to breaking the cycle is to keep your focus on your feelings, not the food. "Instead of blaming potato chips as the evil temptress, first understand why you need the chips. You may not have the power to change what triggered you to want them, whether that's stress at work or a family illness, but once you've identified what you're feeling, you can experiment with alternative, nonfood ways of coping with it," Sass says.

Sass recommends keeping a food log much in the way you keep (or will be keeping) a training log. The same way you write down not just how long you rode but also the conditions and how you felt, jot down the conditions surrounding your eating. "Write down how you were feeling before, during, and after you eat. It will make you aware of your eating patterns," she says. You may crave crunchy, salty snacks when you're frustrated and not even realize it. Once you've identified what triggers your eating, start experimenting with other responses. If a case of the blues sends you to the freezer for ice cream, see if a short spin around the block chases it away.

DRINKS, BARS, AND GELS

Specially engineered foods like sports drinks, energy bars, and gels have a place in every cyclist's life. But use them judiciously. Energy bars, especially, are designed to be very energy dense, which means they pack a large number of calories in every bite. That's great when you're racing and need hundreds of calories quickly. It's not so great when you're riding to lose weight. If you like the convenience of these products, look for lower-(100-to 200-) calorie bars, like those from Luna, Honey Stinger, and PowerBar Pria. Or cut your regular energy bars in half for automatic portion control. You can also find lower-calorie energy drinks like G2 from Gatorade for those days when you need the fluid without the extra carbs and calories.

DROP POUNDS WITH DOWNLOADS

Studies show that people are far more successful at losing weight and keeping it off when they monitor their food intake. Problem is that it can be a drag to carry around a journal and write everything down. Enter the digital age. Now you can keep track via text messaging through any number of free applications available for your phone. Applications like Lose It and Calorie Tracker (available through Livestrong.com) let you create a daily calorie budget, record food and exercise, set goals, and monitor your progress. Some of them even offer a nutritional database that includes hundreds of thousands of restaurant items, so you're always armed with the information you need to make intelligent weight-loss choices.

Whatever you do, don't eat food because you feel guilty about letting it go to waste. What are you really accomplishing by eating those cookies brought over by a neighbor or the leftover Chinese you weren't crazy about the first time? Throwing out food never feels good, but it is not a crime. Gorging on unneeded calories and "waisting" them isn't any better than dispensing of them. It still means we have more food than we need while others have less. Wearing that fact around your middle isn't going to change that or make those with less more appreciative. Sure, we should all try to keep our food waste to a minimum. But don't feel a moral obligation to eat something simply so it doesn't go to waste.

One more thing: Ditch the all-or-nothing thinking once and for all. A bad minute with a bag of Doritos does not have to make a bad day. A bad day does not have to make a bad week. A bad week does not mean you've blown it for life. And none of it means you're a bad person. What matters is the big picture. If you indulge a little more than you planned at one meal or party, just get back on track and eat a little less at the next couple of meals or the next day. This is not a diet. This is not a meal plan that you're going to go on until you lose a certain number of pounds and then abandon for your old ways. This is a complete shift in the way you eat and think about food. Like any change, it will take some time to sink in, but once it does, it will be with you for life, even if it's not always easy, says Elizabeth Potter, the bike rider from Utah who is also a longtime emotional eater.

"Before cycling I ate whatever and whenever I wanted. I self-medicated with food. I ate when I was sad. I ate when I was happy. I ate during all my mood swings. I didn't eat for nutritional reasons. I ate to feel better. However, once I began to exercise and cycle, my dieting changed, dramatically. I started thinking of food as fuel for my riding and concentrated on making healthier choices.

"Food is still a struggle today. I have always eaten emotionally. I found food a comfort. It was never a solution, but it has always been there to temporarily fill my emotions. Food made me feel better about myself. So I had to change my thoughts. Today, before I put food into my mouth I find myself asking myself 'Am I really hungry?' I sometimes think of an apple—if that sounds good and I could eat one, then I know I am hungry. I also always have to think, is this something that is going to help my bike ride the next day, or will it hinder it? I need to fuel my body; I can't eat for fulfillment purposes.

"I am not perfect at all. I am human and I still want chocolate and sweet treats. I will indulge every once in a while, but it's moderation not deprivation. I just have to stay in control when I eat. I know where I can eat and what I can eat."

6: TAKE IT INSIDE

MAKE THOSE RIDES TO "NOWHERE" TAKE YOU SOMEWHERE GREAT

AS I WRITE this, it's 19 degrees outside. Some days I'll brave it and bundle up to ride outside (particularly if I have a few fellow cold-weather cyclists to keep me company). Some days I just can't bear it. On those days, I simply bring my bike inside, put it aboard my indoor trainer or rollers, and listen to my favorite iPod playlists, *This American Life* on NPR, or a special indoor workout podcast that talks me through a 60-minute session including a series of intervals. When I'm done, I feel as if I've really done something . . . because I have really done something. Though indoor riding can't hold a candle to the outdoor experience, it is a powerful training tool that burns a ton of calories.

If you live pretty much anywhere in the Northern Hemisphere, work a job that limits your potential daylight riding time, or generally have a life that sometimes steps in between you and your bike, having indoor riding options will help you keep pedaling while barely missing a beat. In some ways it may even help you get a leg up on your riding fitness.

Because you don't coast, cruise, draft, or really ever stop pedaling when riding indoors, you generally put in more total work per hour than you do when riding outside. Trainers are also very effective for interval workouts, because you never have to worry about being interrupted by a stoplight or traffic. It's also easier to pay attention to the numbers on your computer, because you're not concerned about keeping your eyes on the road (priority number one outside). When you do six 2-minute intervals on your trainer, you know you've done the same work in the same conditions. That makes inside riding pretty strong medicine. In fact, Chris Carmichael (Lance Armstrong's coach) has shown that cyclists can boost their maximum sustainable power output by 12 percent after just 8 weeks of consistent indoor training.

INDOOR OPTIONS

Just as there are any number of bikes to choose from, trainers come in all shapes and sizes, each having its own unique advantages and limitations. Here's a look at the most popular varieties.

Turbo trainers. Most often called simply "trainers," these triangular platforms fasten onto your rear wheel, which rolls along a metal drum, turning your bike into a stationary bike. Trainers range in price from $150 to $450, and just as in bicycles, you do get what you pay for. Cheaper models can be wobbly (I know larger riders who have actually tipped them over), clunky, and extremely noisy (not much fun when you're trying to watch your favorite TV show to pass the time). Higher-end models provide a smoother pedal feel as well as greater stability and blissfully little noise. Because your bike is fixed in place, pedaling will still feel a little unnatural. But newer models do a pretty admirable job of making the action as realistic as possible. You'll find three types of trainers.

Wind. As the name implies, these trainers use air to provide resistance as your back tire spins a roller that's attached to a fan. The nice thing about wind trainers is they closely mimic the resistance of outside riding, as it gets harder to pedal the faster you go. They're very simple systems that tend to be pretty inexpensive and hassle free. The downside is that they can be pretty loud (though newer models are a little less so) and may also vibrate. They usually provide just one resistance level, though you can always shift to make pedaling harder or easier.

Magnetic. Whisper quiet and relatively inexpensive, this type of trainer uses magnets to provide the riding resistance. Problem is that in most models, as you pedal faster, the resistance doesn't get exponentially harder the way it does on the road (or with wind trainers), so the ride feel is less realistic. (CycleOps, however, now sells a progressive resistance magnetic trainer.) Most magnetic trainers counteract this drawback by providing adjustment settings that allow you to manually increase or decrease the resistance.

Fluid. Generally the most expensive of the bunch, fluid trainers are also the quietest and most realistic when it comes to ride quality. Fluid trainers are essentially wind trainers submerged in a silicone fluid that provides the resistance. They generate progressively harder resistance the faster you pedal, just like outside riding. Their one drawback is leakage. The oil inside heats up considerably during hard sessions, and it's possible for the seal that keeps the fluid contained to fail, leaving you with a bit of a mess. Newer models are more secure with less likelihood of failure. Just something to be aware of should you decide to go cruising for a deal on eBay.

Rollers. This type of trainer is a set of three steel drums fixed to a rectangular frame. You take your entire bike, place it on top, hold on to something sturdy to get your balance, and start pedaling. Rollers are an excellent workout, because there is zero downtime on them. To stay upright, you must be pedaling smoothly, consistently, and continuously the entire time. They're great for perfecting pedaling technique and building endurance. They're not very good for interval workouts, however, because you can't perform all-out sprints, stand up, or move around much without the risk of toppling off them. They also require a lot of mental focus, which some riders find more exhausting than the workout itself.

The one exception is Inside Ride E-Motion rollers. They are fixed to a sliding platform surrounded by bumpers. Because they move with you, you can actually stand up, toss your bike around a little, and generally ride as you would outside. They're as close to real riding as I've encountered in a trainer. Of course, such technology does come with a price, and it's on the higher end (they run in the $700 range).

Spin bikes. These are the heavy stationary bikes with the weighted flywheel you see in the gym. You're not likely to shell out a grand or so for one of these (especially given their complete lack of portability), but they do provide a good cycling-specific workout. Some cyclists prefer to take Spinning classes a few times a week during the winter to keep their cycling fitness sharp. Or you can take the workouts provided here and in the programs in Chapter 4 and do your own routine.

INSIDE RIDES

Inside riding is like medicine. A little is great; more is not always better. For one, you'll be bored out of your mind if you try to pull a marathon session of going nowhere. It's also more wearing on you physically. You're not only putting out more effort, you're also generally not moving around as much on your bike, which puts more pressure on your hands, feet, and butt—all of which will be happier if you limit the indoor rides to no more than 90 minutes.

Here is a selection of indoor workouts that will sharpen all elements of your cycling fitness as well as burn fat and build endurance. Each one takes just 45 minutes to an hour to complete and will help the time fly by. You can do these two or three times a week during the off-season. Or use them as supplemental training year-round. You can also do any of the shorter workouts from the four weight-loss plans on your trainer. As a rule of thumb, however, reduce the total riding time by about 20 percent when you take an outdoor workout indoors. So if you were going to ride 75 minutes, shave it down to an hour. Keep the intervals and recovery periods the same length, but reduce the overall ride time.

Base your workouts on the same breathing intensity scale recommended in the plans found in Chapter 4.

Zone 1: Light and relaxed breathing—barely above normal. It's a rate of perceived exertion (RPE) of 1 to 2.

Zone 2: Deep, steady, relaxed breathing. That's your aerobic, endurance-training zone, with an RPE of 3 to 4.

Zone 3: Slightly labored. This is a steady "tempo" pace, where you're working just a hair above your endurance comfort zone. It's where you'd be if you were riding with someone just slightly faster than you. It's an RPE of 5 to 6.

Zone 4: Short, quick, rhythmic breathing. This is your lactate threshold zone, right where you're hitting your sustainable upper limits. Also known as race pace, it's an RPE of 7 to 8.

Zone 5: Hard, gasping-for-breath breathing. This is your VO_2 max training zone, which is a fancy way of saying the top of your limit, as hard as you can go. It's an RPE of 9 to 10.

HEAD FOR THE HILLS

The following three workouts simulate the demands of hilly rides. For these (and any inside rides where you're setting the resistance to high), be wary of excess load on your knees when you're setting the tension on your bike. The work should stress your muscles, not your knee joint. If you are using a Spin bike at the gym, try to adjust the seat height and fore/aft position as close as possible to the measurements of your personal bike.

The 15-minute warmup will be the same for all workouts. It is as follows:

Real Ride Warmup

3 minutes: Spin easy in Zone 1.

2 minutes: Spinups—Zone 1 spin, start with a neutral cadence; Zone 2 spin, slightly quicker than neutral; Zone 3, a little quicker; Zone 4, the quickest spin you can hold.

2 minutes: Repeat spinups, this time with increased resistance.

1 minute: In Zone 2 with three 10-second quick spins followed by recovery.

2 minutes: Climb preparation, Zone 3. Start at a flat resistance that mimics a very slight climb. Every 30 seconds increase your resistance a notch, until you've completed four 30-second segments.

3 minutes: Climb prep, harder resistance, Zones 3 to 4. Start at a resistance that mimics a moderate climb. Increase the resistance every 45 seconds (standing for the first 15 seconds and sitting for the remaining 30 seconds) until you've completed four 45-second segments.

2 minutes: two 30-second VO_2 maximal (Zone 5) efforts, 60-second recovery (Zone 1) in between.

Mountain Assault

Real Ride Warmup

15 minutes (as described on opposite page.)

The Main Event

4 minutes: Seated climb with the bike tension set so you're working in Zone 3.

2 minutes: Easy spinning recovery, Zone 1.

4 minutes: Seated climb, Zone 3; then increase your cadence, finishing the final 30 seconds faster than you started.

2 minutes: Easy spinning recovery, Zone 1.

4 minutes: Seated climb, Zone 3; then increase your cadence, finishing the final 60 seconds faster than you started, increasing the tension and standing and sprinting the last 30 seconds, Zone 4.

2 minutes: Easy spinning recovery, Zone 1.

4 minutes: Seated climb, Zone 3; then increase your cadence, finishing the final 60 seconds faster than you started, increasing the tension and standing and sprinting the last 30 seconds, Zone 4.

2 minutes: Easy spinning recovery, Zone 1.

1 minute: Standing climb, Zone 4.

Cooldown

10 minutes: Easy spinning recovery, Zone 1.

Total time: 50 minutes.

Rock the Rollers

Real Ride Warmup

15 minutes (as described on page 126).

The Main Event

3 minutes: Adjust tension to mimic a hill. Pedal seated at 70 to 80 rpm, keeping pedal stroke smooth and fluid, Zone 3, for 1 minute; increase tension and climb out of the saddle 1 minute; sit back down (keeping tension constant) and push it to the top for 1 minute, ending in Zone 4.

1 minute: Spin at 90+ rpm, Zones 1 to 2.

3 minutes: Adjust tension to mimic a hill. Pedal seated at 70 to 80 rpm, keeping pedal stroke smooth and fluid, Zone 3, for 1 minute; increase tension and climb out of the saddle 1 minute; sit back down (keeping tension constant) and push it to the top for 1 minute, ending in Zone 4.

1 minute: Spin at 90+ rpm, Zones 1 to 2.

3 minutes: Adjust tension to mimic a hill. Pedal seated at 70 to 80 rpm, keeping pedal stroke smooth and fluid, Zone 3, for 1 minute; increase tension and climb out of the saddle 1 minute; sit back down (keeping tension constant) and push it to the top for 1 minute, ending in Zone 4.

3 minutes: Spin at 90+ rpm, Zones 1 to 2.

Repeat main set, using more tension, if possible.

Cooldown

10 minutes: Easy spinning recovery, Zone 1.

Total time: Approximately 55 minutes.

Steep and Surging

Real Ride Warmup

15 minutes (as described on page 126).

The Main Event

2 minutes: Increase resistance so you're climbing at a cadence of 70 rpm, Zone 3.

30 seconds: Accelerate to increase cadence to 80 rpm, Zone 4.

30 seconds: Increase resistance a notch, maintaining your 80-rpm cadence, Zone 4.

15 seconds: Increase resistance one more notch, stand, and accelerate to Zone 5.

5 minutes: Pedal easy at a high cadence above 90 rpm, Zones 1 to 2.

Repeat the sequence above 4 more times.

Cooldown

5 minutes: Easy spinning recovery, Zone 1.

Total time: Approximately 60 minutes.

☀FAST BREAKS

The following three workouts are designed to boost your top-end fitness so you can ride faster and harder. It's important to keep good form during these efforts. If you find yourself flailing, dial back the intensity until your movements are back in control.

Sprint 60s

Real Ride Warmup

15 minutes (as described on page 126).

The Main Event

1 minute: Accelerate until you are working in Zones 4 to 5, nearly as hard as you can go.

2 minutes: Pedal easy at a high cadence above 90 rpm, Zone 2.

Repeat 7 more times for a total of 8 interval/recovery periods.

5 minutes: Pedal at a moderate effort, holding a high cadence (90 rpm), in Zones 2 to 3.

Cooldown

About 10 minutes: Easy spinning recovery, Zone 1.

Total time: Approximately 55 minutes.

Speed Pyramid

Real Ride Warmup

15 minutes (as described on page 126).

The Main Event

90 seconds: Turn up the resistance to the point that it's difficult to spin a high cadence, but not so high that you can't pedal smoothly. Rise out of the saddle and start sprinting. Hold a cadence of 90 to 95 rpm, Zones 4 to 5.

2 minutes: Lower resistance and spin easy, Zones 1 to 2.

75 seconds: Turn up the resistance to the point that it's difficult to spin a high cadence, but not so high that you have to mash. Rise out of the saddle and start sprinting. Hold a cadence of 90 to 95 rpm, Zones 4 to 5.

2 minutes: Lower resistance and spin easy, Zones 1 to 2.

60 seconds: Turn up the resistance to the point that it's difficult to spin a high cadence, but not so high that you have to mash. Rise out of the saddle and start sprinting. Hold a cadence of 90 to 95 rpm, Zones 4 to 5.

2 minutes: Lower resistance and spin easy, Zones 1 to 2.

45 seconds: Turn up the resistance to the point that it's difficult to spin a high cadence, but not so high that you have to mash. Rise out of the saddle and start sprinting. Hold a cadence of 90 to 95 rpm, Zones 4 to 5.

2 minutes: Lower resistance and spin easy, Zones 1 to 2.

30 seconds: Turn up the resistance to the point that it's difficult to spin a high cadence, but not so high that you have to mash. Rise out of the saddle and start sprinting. Hold a cadence of 90 to 95 rpm, Zone 5.

2 minutes: Lower resistance and spin easy, Zones 1 to 2.

15 seconds: Turn up the resistance to the point that it's difficult to spin a high cadence, but not so high that you have to mash. Rise out of the saddle and start sprinting. Hold a cadence of 90 to 95 rpm, Zone 5.

2 minutes: Lower resistance and spin easy, Zones 1 to 2.

30 seconds: Turn up the resistance to the point that it's difficult to spin a high cadence, but not so high that you have to mash. Rise out of the saddle and start sprinting. Hold a cadence of 90 to 95 rpm, Zone 5.

2 minutes: Lower resistance and spin easy, Zones 1 to 2.

45 seconds: Turn up the resistance to the point that it's difficult to spin a high cadence, but not so high that you have to mash. Rise out of the saddle and start sprinting. Hold a cadence of 90 to 95 rpm, Zones 4 to 5.

2 minutes: Lower resistance and spin easy, Zones 1 to 2.

60 seconds: Turn up the resistance to the point that it's difficult to spin a high cadence, but not so high that you have to mash. Rise out of the saddle and start sprinting. Hold a cadence of 90 to 95 rpm, Zones 4 to 5.

2 minutes: Lower resistance and spin easy, Zones 1 to 2.

75 seconds: Turn up the resistance to the point that it's difficult to spin a high cadence, but not so high that you have to mash. Rise out of the saddle and start sprinting. Hold a cadence of 90 to 95 rpm, Zones 4 to 5.

2 minutes: Lower resistance and spin easy, Zones 1 to 2.

90 seconds: Turn up the resistance to the point that it's difficult to spin a high cadence, but not so high that you have to mash. Rise out of the saddle and start sprinting. Hold a cadence of 90 to 95 rpm, Zones 4 to 5.

2 minutes: Lower resistance and spin easy, Zones 1 to 2.

Cooldown

10 to 12 minutes: Easy spinning recovery, Zone 1.

Total time: Approximately 60 minutes.

3-2-1 Blast off

Real Ride Warmup

15 minutes (as described on page 126).

The Main Event

3 minutes: Increase intensity so you're pushing in Zone 4.

2 minutes: Increase intensity again, pushing in Zones 4 to 5.

1 minute: Crank up the intensity, so you finish the final 15 seconds as hard as you can go in Zone 5.

6 minutes: Lower resistance and spin easy, Zones 1 to 2.

Repeat the main set once more from the beginning.

Cooldown

10 minutes: Easy spinning recovery, Zone 1.

Total time: Approximately 50 minutes.

TURN ON THE TEMPO

The following pair of workouts improves your sustainable power and leg strength so you can ride longer, more comfortably at higher speeds and intensities. As always, maintain proper form throughout the entire workout. Adjust the resistance so the effort remains in your muscles, never your joints.

Steady-State Hat Trick

Real Ride Warmup

15 minutes (as described on page 126).

The Main Event

8 to 10 minutes (start with 8 and work up to 10): Steady state—increase your intensity to the upper edges of Zone 3 (if possible) and hold steady there, keeping your pedaling fluid and smooth, upper body relaxed.

5 minutes: Lower intensity and pedal easily, Zone 2.

8 to 10 minutes (start with 8 and work up to 10): Steady state—increase your intensity to the upper edges of Zone 3 (if possible) and hold steady there, keeping your pedaling fluid and smooth, upper body relaxed.

5 minutes: Lower intensity and pedal easily, Zone 2.

8 to 10 minutes (start with 8 and work up to 10): Steady state—increase your intensity to the upper edges of Zone 3 (if possible) and hold steady there, keeping your pedaling fluid and smooth, upper body relaxed.

Cooldown

5 to 10 minutes: Easy spinning recovery, Zone 1.

Total time: Approximately 60 minutes.

Heavy Metal Pedaling

(Skip this drill if you have a history of knee problems.)

Real Ride Warmup

15 minutes (as described on page 126).

The Main Event

5 minutes: Big gear push—increase the resistance so you can just pedal at about 60 rpm in Zones 3 to 4. Though the effort is hard, you should still be able to pedal fluidly, without mashing (or feeling pain in your knees).

5 minutes: Reduce the resistance and increase your cadence to recover in Zones 1 to 2.

Repeat the main set 3 more times for a total of 4 intervals.

(Work up to doing two 15-minute intervals with 10 minutes of recovery.)

Cooldown

5 to 10 minutes: Easy spinning recovery, Zone 1.

Total time: Approximately 60 minutes.

RIDE SIMULATORS

The following workouts from James Herrera, founder of Performance Driven consulting in Colorado Springs, Colorado, simulate the real riding experience, including hard short bursts, longer tempo pushes, easy spinning, and the basic undulating effort you put forth out on the road.

Up and Over

Real Ride Warmup

15 minutes (as described on page 126).

The Main Event

2 minutes: Moderate pedaling, Zone 2.

12 minutes: Over/under threshold efforts—ride 3 minutes in Zone 3, then 1 minute in Zone 4. Repeat 2 more times.

1 minute: Easy spinning recovery, Zone 1.

1 minute: Moderate pedaling, Zone 2.

$10^1/_2$ minutes: Over/under max efforts—ride 3 minutes in Zone 4, then 30 seconds in Zone 5. Repeat 2 more times.

1 minute: Easy spinning recovery, Zone 1.

1 minute: Moderate pedaling, Zone 2.

4 minutes: Progressive climb—increase resistance to mimic a moderate climb (Zone 4), stand and push for 15 seconds, then sit for 45 seconds. Increase resistance, repeating the sequence 3 more times.

Cooldown

5 to 10 minutes: Easy spinning recovery, Zone 1.

Total time: Approximately 40 minutes.

Push It

Real Ride Warmup

15 minutes (as described on page 126).

The Main Event

2 minutes: Moderate pedaling, Zone 2.

2 minutes: Steady brisk pedaling, Zone 3.

12 minutes: Big gear push—increase resistance until you feel as though you're pushing a hard gear. Push 2 minutes, standing the first 30 seconds to get on top of the effort, Zone 4. Recover for 1 minute, pedaling moderately, Zone 2. Repeat 3 more times for a total of 4 intervals.

1 minute: Easy spinning recovery, Zone 1.

1 minute: Moderate pedaling, Zone 2.

8 minutes: Hill surges—increase resistance so you feel as though you're on a moderate to hard climb, but pedaling in a smooth, controlled manner, Zone 3. After 1 minute, increase resistance and accelerate out of the saddle for 20 seconds, Zone 4. Reduce resistance and pedal at a moderate pace for 1 minute, Zone 2. Repeat the surge/recover sequence 5 more times.

1 minute: Easy spinning recovery, Zone 1.

1 minute: Moderate pedaling, Zone 2.

10 minutes: Full-on sprint. Crank up your pace as hard as you can go for 2 minutes, Zone 5. Ease off to easy recovery pace for 2 minutes, Zone 1. Repeat 2 more times for a total of 3 intervals.

Cooldown

5 to 10 minutes: Easy spinning recovery, Zone 1.

Total time: Approximately 60 minutes.

Off to the Races

Real Ride Warmup

15 minutes (as described on page 126).

The Main Event

2 minutes: Moderate pedaling, Zone 2.

6 minutes: Steady-state effort, Zone 3—increase your resistance so you feel as though you're in a slightly big gear or on an incline. Stand for 30 seconds, pedal seated for 1 minute. Repeat 3 more times for a total of 4 intervals.

9 minutes: Over/under threshold efforts—increase resistance and accelerate so you're working hard in Zone 4 for 2 minutes. Reduce intensity and pedal moderately in Zone 2 for 1 minute. Repeat 2 more times for a total of 3 intervals.

1 minute: Easy spinning recovery, Zone 1.

1 minute: Moderate pedaling, Zone 2.

20 minutes: Race 5 minutes at hard effort, Zones 4 to 5, followed by $2^1/_2$ minutes of very easy pedaling, Zone 1. Repeat 2 more times.

Cooldown

5 minutes: Easy spinning recovery, Zone 1.

Total time: Approximately 60 minutes.

❉SET YOURSELF UP TO SUCCEED

At some point, just about all of us have bought some piece of exercise equipment that was supposed to revolutionize our workouts, but soon became relegated to a dusty corner to play the role of a $500 coat rack. That usually happens for two reasons: (1) It's a pain in the neck to set up; (2) you're bored with it, so it's not worth setting up. Don't let that happen to your bicycling trainer. The key to keeping momentum is to make indoor riding convenient and enjoyable.

Start by setting up your trainer in a pleasant spot. I can't tell you how many times I've had clients complain that they just can't drag themselves onto the trainer. Then when I go to their house, I see a lone bike set up in the gloomiest, dankest basement corner. No surprise that you're not going to be chomping at the bit to head down to a dungeon environment in the dead of winter. I place my rollers by the window in our laundry room. I can play music while I spin and watch the snow fall. It's actually kind of lovely. It's also out of the way enough so I can leave it set up all winter long. That's important, because if I had to drag out my rollers every time I wanted to ride, I would ride far less.

Stock your space with a television, iPod dock, or other entertainment of your choice. Unless it's a cool room in the house, you'll also want a fan and a towel. It's surprising how much sweat you drip when it's not being whooshed away by the passing breeze. One thing that works for me is keeping some pre-programmed playlists on my iPod. Even when I am absolutely not feeling like spinning my wheels to nowhere, I push Play and the first few strains of AC/DC's "Girls Got Rhythm" or "Boom Boom Pow" by the Black Eyed Peas is guaranteed to lift my spirits and make my legs move. You even can arrange your playlist to mimic an outside ride. Here's an example:

Warmup. Energetic tune to perk you up and get your body moving (i.e., "Music" by Madonna).

Flat and fast. High-tempo song to inspire a little speed (i.e., "Pump It" by the Black Eyed Peas).

Sustained climb. Steady, slower rhythm for a moderate to hard climb (i.e., "Temperature" by Sean Paul).

Downhill. High-speed pedaling. Fast and furious (i.e., "Girls Got Rhythm" by AC/DC).

Steady-state effort. Churning at a brisk (90 rpm) cadence under moderate resistance (i.e., "Days Go By" by Dirty Vegas).

Cruising. Easy spinning for a few minutes of recovery (i.e., "All Because of You" by U2).

Steep climb. Hard-driving, slow-tempo beat (i.e., "Lose Yourself" by Eminem).

Flat and fast. High-energy song to spin out your legs (i.e., "The Fame" by Lady GaGa).

Sprints to the finish. Fast-driving tune to finish with two to three 30-second sprints (i.e., "Freestyle Noize" by the Freestylers).

Cooldown. Easy, happy cruising music to let your heart rate come down (i.e., "No Rain" by Blind Melon).

It's that simple. Before you know it, another workout will be in the books, and you'll be one step closer to realizing your weight-loss goals.

7: OFF-THE-BIKE TRAINING

REV YOUR METABOLISM, GET STRONGER, RIDE FASTER, HAVE MORE FUN

NOTHING BEATS RIDING a bike. But realistically, most of us can't ride every day year-round. Work, life, weather, and sometimes general lack of motivation can knock you out of the saddle for a few days. That's completely natural. In fact, it's healthy.

Time spent doing other activities like strength-training, stretching, and cross-training will help you stay mentally fresh and will also give you more balanced fitness than if you did nothing but bike alone. Here's a look at some cross-training activities that will complement your cycling and weight-loss efforts and a rundown on how to make them work for you.

⁂STRENGTH-TRAINING: STRONG CYCLISTS STAY LEAN AND HEALTHY

For years strength-training and cycling "enjoyed" a sort of oil and water relationship. You could mix them if you tried hard enough, but they invariably would end up separating again. Top-level cyclists (and their coaches) simply worried that any kind of resistance-training would bulk them up and slow them down. Today, a fair number of pros in even the most distinguished pelotons devote at least some of their season to strength-training. Many coaches now recognize that making some lean muscle is a big help rather than a hindrance to most recreational riders. This is especially true for riders looking to lose weight.

"When you're overweight, especially if you're extremely overweight, it's hard to do long bouts of cardio exercise like long bike rides," says Brian Strauser, who lost more than 100 pounds by lifting weights in his apartment and riding every day. Anyone can lift weights, and it helps to build muscle and be stronger to do everything else. Having strong, well-toned muscles means better balance and bike handling and less fatigue (which can take the form of back and neck aches) on the road. It also increases your stamina, both mentally and physically. "Physically, it allows your body to pedal longer and harder and for your arms and shoulders to support you longer without getting tired," he says. "Having more strength allows you to be mentally prepared when heading out there so that you can handle anything."

More lean tissue also burns more calories—a must for people looking to lose weight. Muscle is the engine that keeps your metabolism burning high. Unfortunately, it's hard to hold on to. Sometime after you blow out the candles on your 30th birthday cake, your metabolism slows down to the tune of 5 percent a decade—a seemingly small decline, until you figure that it can add up to more than 10 unwanted pounds a year. And it's muscle loss that is mostly to blame for this metabolism meltdown. "After 30 you start losing 5 pounds of muscle per decade," says Wayne Westcott, PhD, CSCS, fitness research director at the South Shore YMCA in Quincy, Massachusetts. "When muscle mass diminishes, so does your calorie-burning ability. You end up replacing that lost lean tissue with fat—up to twice as much," he says. With less muscle, you're also less strong, so everything from walking upstairs to playing with your kids is more tiring. So you move less, and gain more.

There's been much debate over how many calories muscle tissue versus fat tissue burns, but most researchers agree that muscle is far more metabolically active, using up about five times as many calories at rest as fat does (plus nice, toned muscles also look better on the beach, but that's another story). What may be more important in the weight-loss equation is that, as Brian was so quick to realize, more muscle means more strength and more energy. In short, when you're stronger and fitter, you're more likely to burn more calories when you're out riding and generally living your life.

Speaking of strength, cycling, as you learned earlier, is a power-to-weight sport. The more power you can produce per pound of body weight, the faster you'll fly up hills and hammer down the road. We're already working on the weight side of the equation. Now let's get busy pumping up the power end. Pushing your pedals, especially against gravity or other elements like wind, takes a lot of power, which by definition is the ability to do lots of work in a short amount of time. You need strength—the ability to move your weight as well as your bike's weight—to have power. Resistance-training activates sleeping muscle fibers, bolsters those that are currently weak, and helps build more to do the work you want to do—that means stronger muscles that will allow you to produce more power on the bike. But the ability to push harder into your pedals is just one (and maybe not even the most important) way resistance-training can make you a stronger cyclist.

Riding a bike takes far more than strong legs. Watch a pro cycling race on TV sometime. The first sign of riders who have "cracked," meaning they're too fatigued to ride hard, isn't in their legs. It's in their upper body. They're rocking back and forth on the saddle, sagging through their shoulders and collapsed from their core. Though cycling is a lower-body-dominated sport, your legs don't pedal in isolation. Think of your body as a bike frame. It has to be strong the whole way around to keep you rolling down the road. Any weakness or cracks, and you'll falter. With each revolution, your upper body acts as a platform for your legs to push off of. The more solid your core (abs, obliques, and back muscles), the more power you can deliver into your pedal stroke. The same goes for your arms and shoulders. Sure, they perform the very important function of holding the bar, braking, and steering. But they also help you leverage power as you pull on the bar on an uphill or fast sprint. That power transfers through your core and into your working legs. The stronger the whole chain is, the better (and longer) you can ride without tiring out. That's why even cyclists who shy away from leg presses and lower body training make sure they do core exercises to keep their supporting muscles strong.

Finally, cycling is a non-weight-bearing sport, which is a fancy way of saying that you're not literally pounding the ground with your body weight when you do it. That's great news for people who are carrying extra weight and whose joints groan and moan during impact activities. But it may be less good for your bones, which need a little impact to trigger the bone-remodeling sequence that keeps your bone tissue turning over new cells and staying dense and strong. Most casual cyclists don't have to stress too much over this lack of skeletal impact, but there's enough research pointing to lower bone density in even recreationally competitive cyclists who don't cross-train to make it worthwhile to mention here. The good news is it doesn't take much to get your bones to remodel, and strength-training is one of the best ways to make your muscles and bones strong.

✳MOVES YOU CAN USE TO LOSE

The exercises included in the *Ride Your Way Lean* strength plan are not your typical get-big-muscles Gold's Gym moves. You won't find bicep curls or six moves to isolate every sinew in your shoulders. What you will find are highly functional multimuscle moves that are designed to strengthen your muscles the way your body moves both on and off the bike. I put a special emphasis on core strengthening moves because strong core muscles are the foundation of great performance, no matter what you're doing. As a vanity bonus, because this program emphasizes toning through your abs, back, and obliques, you'll notice that you look 5 to 10 pounds thinner almost immediately because you're standing straighter (strong core muscles help you sit and stand straight and tall), and your belly really will be pulled in a little tighter from strengthening the deep abdominal muscles that wrap around your waist and act as a natural corset for your torso.

The *Ride Your Way Lean* strength plan progresses through three levels: Basic, Intermediate, and Advanced. No matter your weight, weight-loss goals, or cycling experience, you should start at the Basic level. These 10 moves form the strength foundation you'll build on for the next 9 to 12 weeks. Just because the moves are basic doesn't mean they should be easy. They should be challenging. So the weight you select for moves that require dumbbells should be heavy enough that the final repetitions are challenging, but not so heavy that you're not able to maintain balance or proper form. As you get stronger, the moves will feel easier. When you can easily perform all the repetitions in a set (and maybe a few more), it's time to increase the weight. You may find that you need to lower the weight again when you progress to the next level, because the moves themselves present fresh challenges.

As far as equipment goes, you'll need two sets of dumbbells—one set for upper body moves and a heavier set for lower body moves. You'll also need a stability ball. Both of these items are available (and perfectly fine to buy) at most big-box stores. (For more information on strength-training equipment, see "What Else You Need" on page 33.)

Do 12 repetitions of each exercise (unless otherwise indicated), then move immediately to the next move. When you finish the routine, start from the top and perform the entire routine one more time. The whole workout should take no more than about 20 minutes. By doing the moves "circuit" style—that is, straight through with no rest—you will raise your heart rate into an aerobic zone, which improves your overall fitness along with your muscle strength and endurance, and you'll burn more calories to boot. Perform each level for 6 to 8 weeks, then move to the next level.

For each move, you'll find a "Personalize it" option that will alter the move if you find that for reasons of flexibility, strength, balance, or body shape you can't perform the move as recommended with proper form. Do your strength-training routine 2 or 3 days a week, leaving a day between workouts for your muscles to recover. You can piggyback this workout with your hard rides for an extra-tough day or do it before an easy ride, so you can spin out your legs to bring in fresh, nutrient-filled blood, flush out the metabolic waste, and recover even faster from the strength work.

 ## THE BASICS

The best part of these moves is that you don't need to join a gym or invest in any expensive equipment. All you need is your own body and a few basic items, and you'll never have to leave your house or elbow your way through a crowded weight room for a good workout. No hassle and more importantly, no excuses.

Concentrate on performing the moves with good form, lifting deliberately and focusing your attention on firing the muscles that are supposed to be doing the work.

PERFECT PLANK

MUSCLES WORKED: Core and shoulders

Lie facedown on the floor with your upper body propped on your forearms and your elbows directly beneath your shoulders. Your feet should be about hip width apart and propped up on your toes. Contract your abs and lift your body off the floor so your body forms a straight line from your head to your heels, supported by your forearms and toes. Your back should not arch or droop. Hold 10 to 20 seconds, working your way up to 30 seconds. Do 3 repetitions.

Personalize it: If you can't perform this move with bent arms, perform it with your arms extended, hands directly beneath shoulders, as if you were in the "up" position of a pushup.

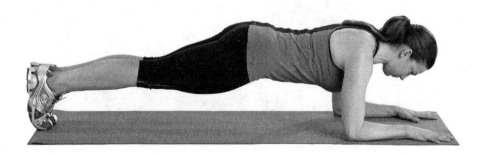

HIP BRIDGE

Lie faceup on the floor with your knees bent 90 degrees and feet flat on the
floor. Squeeze a rolled-up towel between your knees. Pull your navel toward
your spine, contract your glutes, and lift your hips toward the ceiling until
your body forms a straight line from your knees to your shoulders. Lift your
toes so just your heels are on the floor. Pause, and then lower your hips
toward the floor without touching it. Repeat.

Personalize it: Make the move slightly less challenging by keeping
your feet flat on the floor and allowing your body to rest on the floor for a
second between reps.

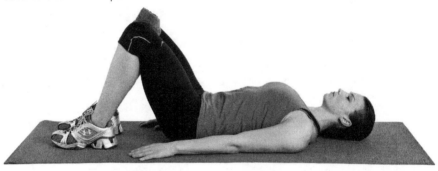

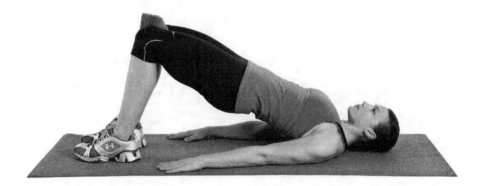

STEPUP

Holding dumbbells in each hand, palms facing in, stand facing a bench or a high step or box (about 12 inches tall). Place your left foot on the bench. Keeping your abs tight and back straight and tall, press into your left foot and lift your body up to a standing position, tapping the bench with your right toes. Keeping your left foot planted, slowly lower back to the starting position. Repeat for a full set. Then switch legs.

Personalize it: Come all the way down to the floor with both feet between repetitions.

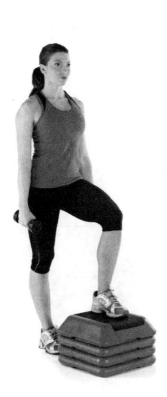
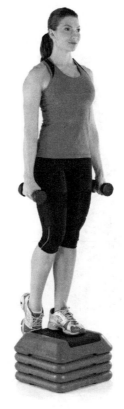

HANDS-UP SQUAT

MUSCLES WORKED: Glutes, hamstrings, and quadriceps

Stand with your feet hip width apart. Place your hands behind your head, elbows bent and pointed out to the sides. Keeping your head up, shoulders back, and back straight, bend your hips and knees as if sitting in a chair. Shift your body weight back into your heels, sticking your butt out as you lower toward the floor. Lower yourself as far as possible while maintaining good form, but don't go lower than 90 degrees, with your thighs parallel to the floor. Keep your knees behind your toes (if you look down you should be able to see your toes). Pause. Then straighten legs and stand back up.

Personalize it: Start with your arms at your sides and bring them straight out in front of you as you lower (so they're parallel to the floor) for balance.

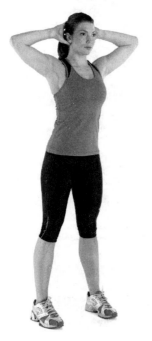

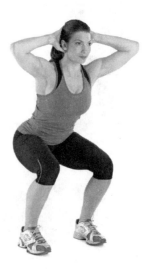

BIRD DOG

MUSCLES WORKED: Back, shoulders, and glutes

Kneel on all fours, with your hands directly beneath your shoulders and knees directly beneath your hips. Keep your back straight and your head in line with your spine. Simultaneously raise your left arm and right leg, extending them in line with your back so your fingers are pointing straight ahead and toes are pointing back. Hold this position for a second. Return to the starting position, and repeat with the opposite arm and leg. That's 1 rep.

Personalize it: If balance is a challenge, start by extending your leg first, then your arm second, rather than moving both at the same time.

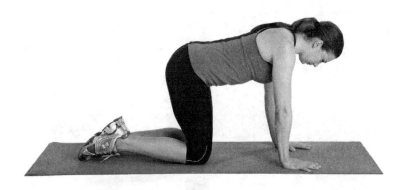

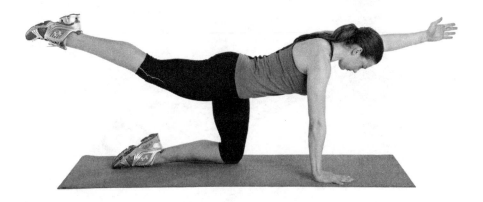

SWISS BALL PUSHUP

MUSCLES WORKED: Chest, shoulders, triceps, and core

Lie facedown on an inflated stability ball with both hands on the floor. Walk your hands out, allowing the ball to roll beneath your body until the ball is under your shins. Your hands should be directly below your shoulders, so it looks as if you're ready to do a pushup. Keeping your torso straight and abs contracted, bend your elbows and lower your chest toward the floor. Stop when your upper arms are parallel to the floor. Pause, and return to the starting position.

Personalize it: The farther you walk your body out on the ball, the more difficult the move becomes. To ease into it, start with the ball underneath your thighs first. Then, as you become more comfortable, gradually walk your hands out farther.

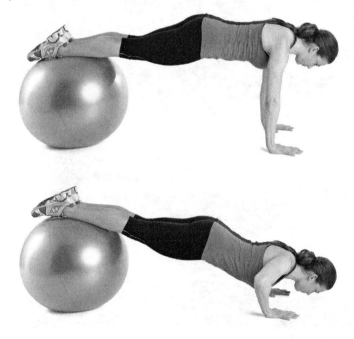

BENT-OVER ROW

MUSCLES WORKED: Back, shoulders, and biceps

Grasp a dumbbell with each hand. Stand with your legs hip width apart and your arms hanging in front of you, palms facing your thighs. Hinge forward at your hips, keeping your back straight and your knees slightly bent. Slowly pull the dumbbells up toward your body until they're at either side of your chest with your elbows pointing toward the ceiling. Pause, and then lower the weights back to the starting position.

Personalize it: Do the move one arm at a time with support. Grasp a dumbbell with your right hand. Bend at the waist and support your weight by putting your left knee and hand on a bench (or the seat of a sturdy chair) so that your back is parallel to the floor. Let your right arm hang straight down with your palm facing the bench. Pull the dumbbell up to your chest, and then lower. Repeat with the other side.

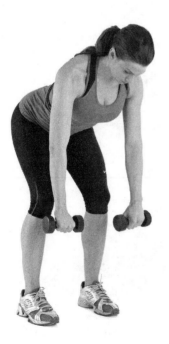 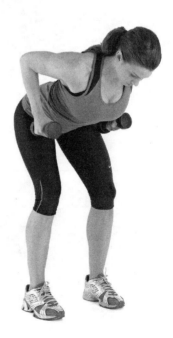

WINDSHIELD WIPER

MUSCLES WORKED: Core

Lie on your back with your knees bent and feet off the floor so your thighs are perpendicular and calves are parallel to the floor. Extend your arms out to the sides, palms facing down. Keeping your shoulders on the floor, slowly drop your legs to the left until they touch the floor. Return to the starting position. Repeat to the opposite side.

Personalize it: Lower your legs only 45 degrees to either side.

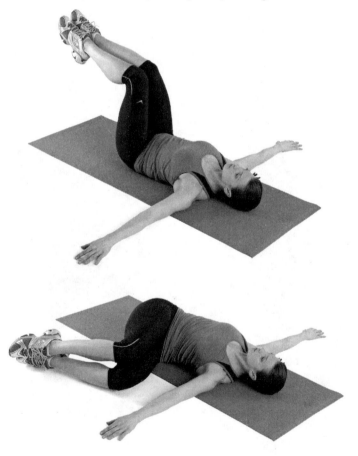

OVERHEAD PRESS

MUSCLES WORKED: Shoulders and upper back

Stand with your feet hip width apart. Hold the dumbbells at shoulder height, palms facing forward. Press the dumbbells straight up overhead and lower back to shoulder height. Don't arch your back.

Personalize it: Perform the move while seated.

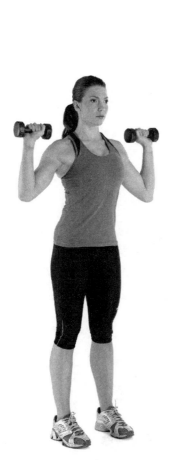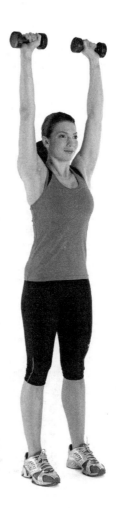

CHAIR DIP

MUSCLES WORKED: Triceps and upper back

Sit on the edge of a sturdy chair, with your hands grasping the seat of the chair at either side of your rear. Walk your feet out slightly and inch your butt off the chair. Extend one leg, so the heel is resting on the floor. Keeping your shoulders down and your back straight, bend your elbows back, and lower your butt toward the floor as far as comfortably possible. Slowly push back up.

Personalize it: Keep both knees bent and feet flat on the floor throughout the move.

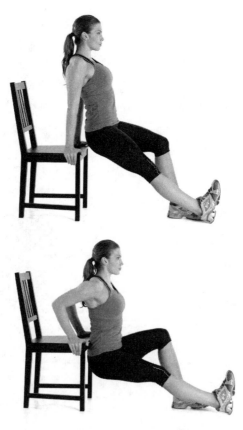

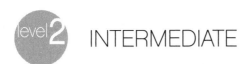

INTERMEDIATE

This Intermediate-level plan takes the Basic moves to the next level by adding a twist to make them more challenging. As before, perform each move slowly and deliberately, concentrating on maintaining good form and firing all the proper muscles.

BELLY-BLASTING PLANK

MUSCLES WORKED: Core, hips, and shoulders

Lie facedown on the floor with your upper body propped on your forearms and your elbows directly beneath your shoulders. Your feet should be about hip width apart and propped up on your toes. Contract your abs and lift your body off the floor so your body forms a straight line from your head to your heels, supported by your forearms and toes. Your back should not arch or droop. Hold this plank position for 10 seconds. Then, tighten your abs and lift your butt toward the ceiling. Hold 5 seconds. Lower to the starting position, and repeat. Do 3 reps.

Personalize it: As before, perform the move with extended arms if you need to in order to create a straight plank off the floor from your head to your heels.

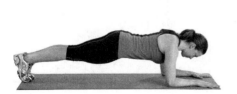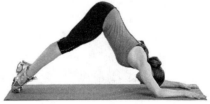

RIDE YOUR WAY LEAN

BRIDGE ON STABILITY BALL

MUSCLES WORKED: Glutes, hips, hamstrings, and core

Lie faceup on the floor with your knees bent 90 degrees and feet flat on a stability ball. Place a rolled-up towel between your knees. Press into the ball with your feet and push your hips into the air so your body forms a straight line from your shoulders to your bent knees. Return to the starting position.

Personalize it: If stability is a problem, perform the move with your feet propped up on a sturdy chair.

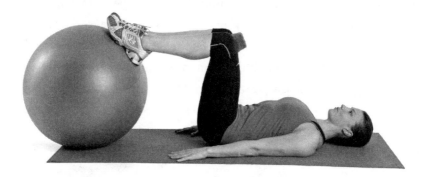

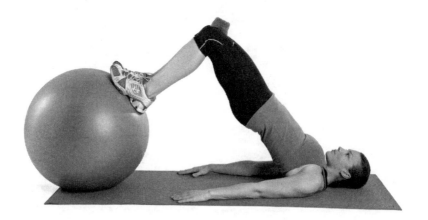

SIDE STEPUP

MUSCLES WORKED: Glutes, hamstrings, quads, adductors (inner thighs), and abductors (outer thighs)

Stand to the side of a box or bench (about 18 inches high). Step up to the top of the box with your right leg, putting your foot on the far right side of the box. Push with your right leg and bring your left foot up next to your right one. Step down to the starting position. Complete a full set, then switch legs.

Personalize it: Use a lower step.

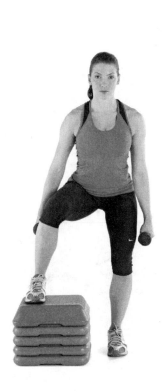
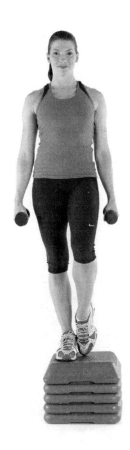

DUMBBELL SQUAT

Stand with your feet hip width apart, holding dumbbells up at your shoulders, palms facing forward. Keeping your head up, shoulders back, and back straight, bend your hips and knees as if sitting in a chair. Shift your body weight back into your heels, sticking your butt out as you lower yourself. Don't go lower than the point where your thighs are parallel to the floor. Keep your knees behind your toes (if you look down, you should be able to see your toes). Pause. Then straighten your legs and stand back up.

Personalize it: Hold the weights down at your sides throughout the move.

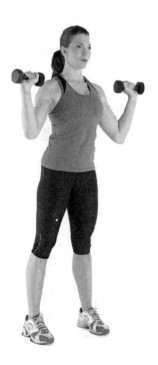
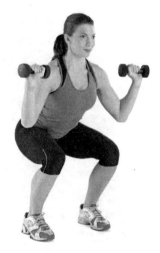

SPIDER

Holding a light dumbbell in each hand, kneel on all fours with your back straight, hands directly beneath your shoulders (weights should run parallel with your body) and knees directly beneath your hips. Simultaneously raise your left arm straight out to the left side while lifting your bent right leg out to the right side. Return to the starting position. Repeat on the opposite side. That's 1 rep.

Personalize it: Perform it without the weights.

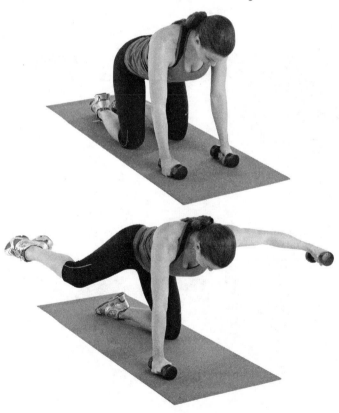

STABILITY BALL JACKKNIFE

MUSCLES WORKED: Core, hips, and glutes

Lie facedown on an inflated stability ball with both hands on the floor. Walk your hands out, allowing the ball to roll beneath your body until the ball is under your ankles and the tops of your feet. Your hands should be directly below your shoulders. Press into the ball, bending your knees and drawing them forward, so you bring your legs and the ball under your torso. Inhale and uncoil as you press back to the starting position.

Personalize it: The farther you walk your body out from the ball, the more difficult the move becomes. Ease into it by starting with the ball under your shins, closer to your knees.

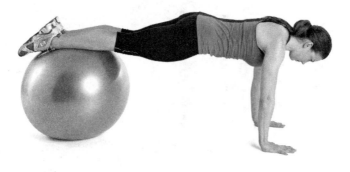

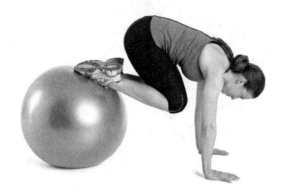

PLANK ROW

MUSCLES WORKED: Core, triceps, shoulders, lats, and biceps

Assume a pushup position with your hands holding the handles of two dumbbells so the weights run parallel to your body. Position your feet hip to shoulder distance apart (the farther apart they are, the easier the move). Keeping your back straight, pull the right dumbbell to your right shoulder, while pressing the left dumbbell into the floor for balance. Return to the starting position and repeat on the other side. Alternate for a full set.

Personalize it: To make the move easier, perform it from your knees, ankles crossed.

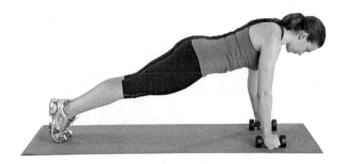

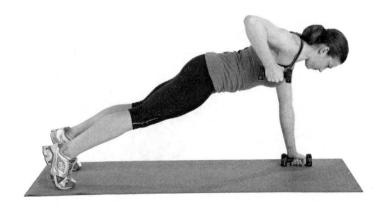

ROCK THE BOAT

MUSCLES WORKED: Core

Sit holding a dumbbell in each hand, with your knees bent and feet flat on the floor. Contract your abs and lift your heels about a foot off the floor, keeping your feet flexed. Lean back so your torso is at about a 45-degree angle with the floor, with the weight suspended directly above your hips. Rotate your upper body to the left and stop when the weight is a few inches from the floor. Hold. Return to the starting position. Repeat to the opposite side. That's 1 rep.

Personalize it: If balance is a challenge, keep your feet planted on the floor.

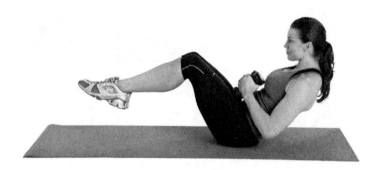

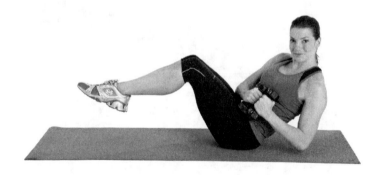

ALTERNATING
OVERHEAD PRESS

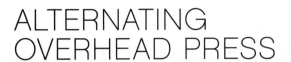

MUSCLES WORKED: Shoulders, upper back, and core

Stand with your feet hip width apart. Hold the dumbbells at shoulder height, palms facing forward. Tighten your abs for stability and press your left arm overhead while keeping your right arm in place. Lower the left arm back to the starting position. Then press the right arm overhead. Return the right arm to the starting position. Continue alternating for a full set on each side.

Personalize it: Perform the move while sitting.

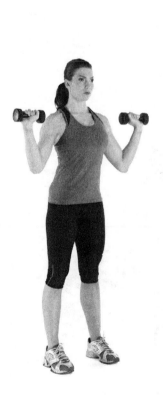
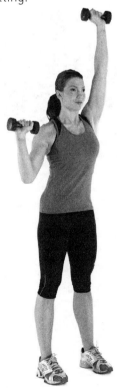

DIP KICK

MUSCLES WORKED: Triceps, core, and quads

Sit on the edge of a chair, with your hands grasping the chair on either side of your hips. Keep your knees bent, with your feet flat on the floor. Scoot your butt off the chair seat. Bend your elbows and lower your hips toward the floor until your upper arms are parallel to the floor. Straighten your arms, lifting your torso upward to the starting position. Once in the up position, extend your right leg straight out. Return to the starting position and repeat with the opposite leg, alternating throughout, for a full set.

Personalize it: Perform the move without the kick.

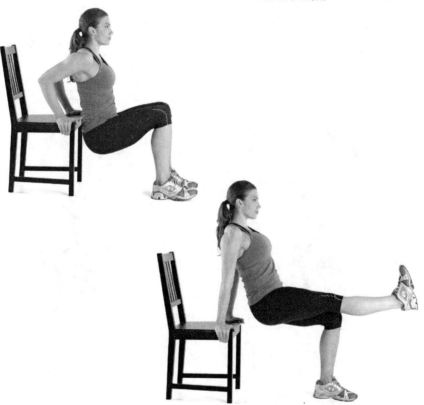

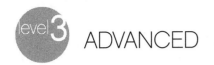 ADVANCED

Once again, you'll take the 10 essential moves and ramp up the difficulty level. This routine is guaranteed to tighten up those core muscles and greatly improve your balance. As before, perform each move slowly and deliberately, concentrating on maintaining good form and firing all the proper muscles.

ONE-ARM PLANK

MUSCLES WORKED: Core, shoulders, and upper back

Lie facedown on the floor with your upper body propped on your forearms and your elbows directly beneath your shoulders. Your feet should be about hip width apart and propped up on your toes. Contract your abs and lift your body off the floor so your body forms a straight line from your head to your heels, supported by your forearms and toes. Your back should not arch or droop. From this position, lift your left arm overhead and out to the side in a half-Y position. Do not allow your body to lean. Hold for 2 seconds. Repeat on the opposite side. Alternate for 6 to 10 lifts per side.

Personalize it: Place your feet wider apart if you can't perform the move without leaning.

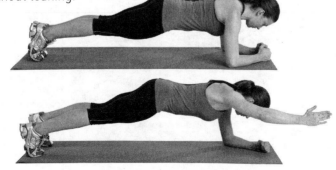

BALL BRIDGE

MUSCLES WORKED: Core, glutes, and quads

Lie back on a stability ball, so it supports your head, shoulders, and upper back. Place your hands behind your head and position your feet close together. Tighten your glutes and raise your hips so your body forms a straight line from your shoulders to your knees with your knees bent 90 degrees. Holding your body stable, extend your right leg with your foot flexed. Pause, lower back to the starting position, and switch legs. That's 1 rep.

Personalize it: If stability is a problem, place your feet shoulder width apart.

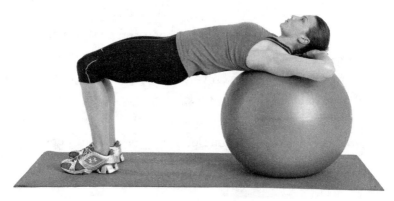

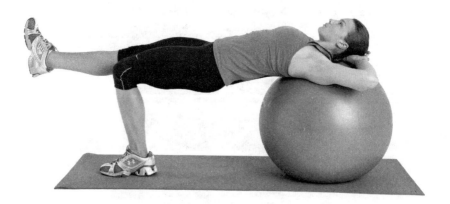

STABILITY BALL PUSH AND PIKE

MUSCLES WORKED: Core, hips, shoulders, and glutes

Lie facedown on an inflated stability ball with both hands on the floor. Walk your hands out, allowing the ball to roll beneath your body until the ball is under your ankles and the tops of your feet. Your hands should be directly below your shoulders. Tighten your abs, lift your hips toward the ceiling, and pull the ball toward your hands with your feet. Keep your legs extended and raise your butt until your body forms an inverted V. Pause, then lower back to the starting position.

Personalize it: The farther you walk your body out from the ball, the more difficult the move becomes. To ease into it, start with the ball underneath your thighs first. Then, as you become more comfortable, gradually walk your hands out farther.

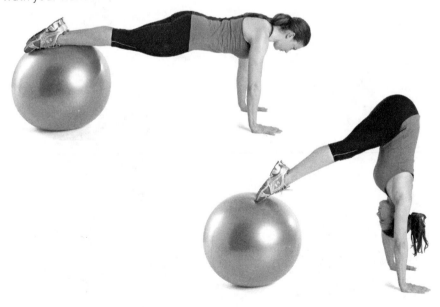

SINGLE-LEG STEPDOWN

MUSCLES WORKED: Glutes, quads, and hamstrings

Holding dumbbells, stand on an 18-inch step with only the left foot on top of the step, allowing the other leg to hang in the air. Pull your navel toward your spine and, keeping your chest lifted, slowly step down with the right foot and gently tap the right heel on the floor. Keeping the left heel firmly planted on the step, return to the starting position. Complete a full set, then switch legs.

Personalize it: Use a shorter (i.e., 12-inch) step if the move is too challenging.

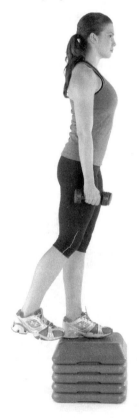
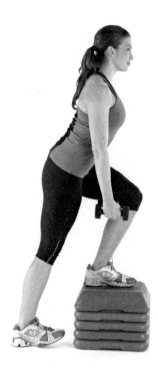

SCOOP SQUAT

MUSCLES WORKED: Glutes, hamstrings,
quadriceps, shoulders, triceps, and core

Holding the weights down at your sides, palms facing your thighs, stand
with your feet hip to shoulder width apart. In one smooth motion, bend
your knees and hips and drop your butt back as though sitting in a chair.
Immediately push back to the starting position, bending your elbows and
curling the weights to your shoulders as you do. As you reach the standing
position, immediately press the weights overhead. Lower the weights back
to your sides and repeat.

Personalize it: Keep the weights at your shoulders without pushing
them overhead if you find yourself arching or swaying. Work up to the overhead press.

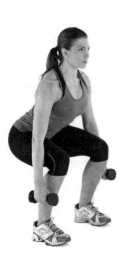
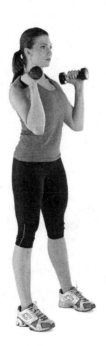
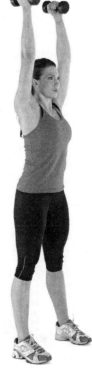

SUSPENDED SUPERMAN

MUSCLES WORKED: Core, upper back, and glutes

Lie facedown on top of a stability ball, so your belly button is at the top of the ball and your hands and feet are on the floor supporting you. Keep your head in line with your back. Contract your glutes and upper-back muscles and raise your left arm and right leg, so they form a straight line parallel to the floor. Pause, lower to the starting position, and repeat on the opposite side.

Personalize it: Perform the move lying facedown on a carpeted floor or mat if you can't achieve the proper position on a stability ball.

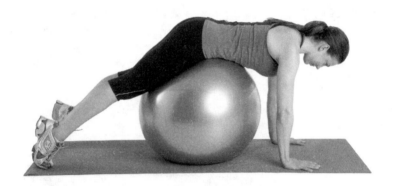

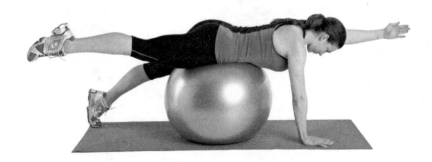

MERMAID

Sit on your right hip with your legs extended to the side, knees slightly bent. Cross your left foot in front of the right. Place your right hand on the floor directly beneath your shoulder. Place your left hand on your left leg. Lift your hips off the floor, extending your left arm overhead, so your body forms a diagonal line. Without bending the right arm, lower your hips and left arm back to the starting position. Repeat for 6 repetitions. Switch sides.

Personalize it: Start with your supporting arm bent, so you are propped on the forearm.

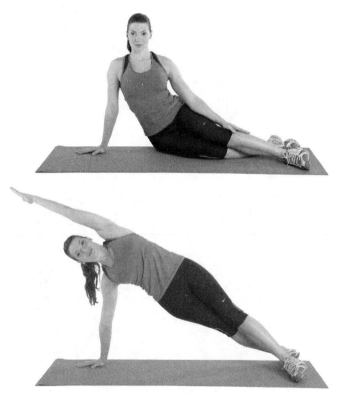

T ROW

MUSCLES WORKED: Glutes, core, back, shoulders, and biceps

Holding dumbbells at your sides, palms facing in, stand with your feet hip to shoulder width apart. Lift your right leg behind you and simultaneously hinge at the hips and drop your upper body forward (keeping your back straight) until your body forms a straight line from head to raised heel and is parallel to the floor, arms hanging toward the floor, palms facing each other. Bend your elbows and pull the weights up to either side of your chest. Lower your arms and then come to the standing position. Repeat on the opposite side. Alternate for a full set.

Personalize it: Lightly hold on to the back of a chair or tabletop for balance with the free hand, if needed.

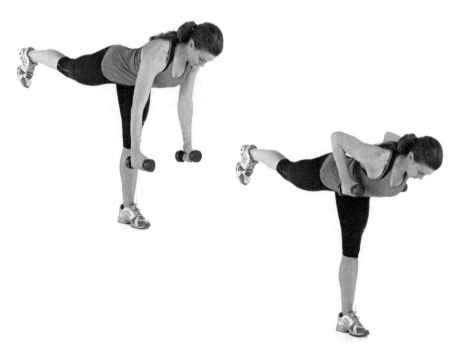

OVERHEAD PRESS WITH TWIST

MUSCLES WORKED: Shoulders, upper back, and core

Stand with your feet hip width apart. Holding a dumbbell in each hand, bend your elbows so the weights are up at your collarbones, facing your body. Tighten your abs, rotate your hands outward, and press your arms overhead so, at the top of the move, your palms are facing forward. Reverse the move, rotating your hands and lowering the weights back to the starting position.

Personalize it: Perform the move while seated if you find yourself arching or swaying.

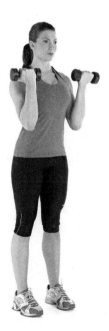
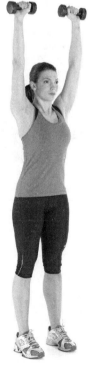

BALANCE DIP AND EXTEND

MUSCLES WORKED: Triceps, quadriceps, upper back, shoulders, and core

Sit on the edge of a chair, with your hands grasping the chair on either side of your hips. Keep your knees bent, with your feet flat on the floor. Scoot your butt off the chair seat. Bend your elbows and lower your hips toward the floor until your upper arms are parallel to the floor. Straighten your arms, then reach your left arm straight out in front of your body at shoulder height, palm facing down, while simultaneously extending your right leg with the foot flexed. Pause. Then bring the arm and leg back to the starting position. Repeat the entire sequence with the other arm and leg. That's 1 rep.

Personalize it: Lift your leg first, then your arm, gradually working up to doing both simultaneously.

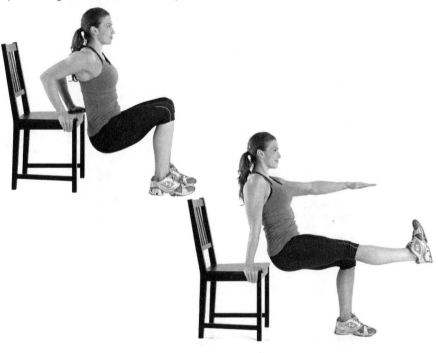

✳STRETCH IT OUT

After sieving through decades of scientific studies and research, the Centers for Disease Control and Prevention (CDC) recently made a startling proclamation: Stretching before exercise does squat for preventing injuries. But before you wave a long-distance good-bye to your toes, take note: The research the CDC was reviewing was on acute injuries—pulls, strains, tears, and sprains—not nagging, painful, sometimes chronic conditions like tendonitis that can be brought on by long-term tightness. If you're going to cycle and strength-train, you should also stretch.

When you stretch, especially the muscles around key cycling joints like your knees and hips, you increase your range of motion, which allows you to generate more power in each pedal stroke to be more balanced and fluid on the bike. You'll also avoid very common cycling aches and pains like iliotibial (IT) band syndrome (pain in the hips and/or knees that results from tightness in the band of tissue running between those joints) or piriformis syndrome (a common cause of sciatica pain), which is the result of the small piriformis muscle in your glutes getting tight and putting pressure on the sciatic nerve. You'll also reverse the Quasimodo-ish forward-flexed syndrome that cyclists can succumb to from being hunched over their bar for hours on end. With your chest more open and shoulders back, you'll be able to breathe easier, climb stronger, and pedal more freely in any position.

The following is a flexibility routine that borrows from yoga and Pilates and focuses on stretching and lengthening the muscles that can get tight and short during cycling. Like all stretches, these are best done when your muscles are warm, such as post cycling. If you do them cold (like in front of your favorite must-see TV in the evening), just ease into them and allow your muscles to warm up as you go.

Some of these stretches are dynamic, meaning you move throughout them. Others are static, meaning you hold them while taking full, even breaths. Perform each stretch for the prescribed repetitions or amount of time. Then move on to the next stretch. If you tend to be particularly tight, go through the routine twice. You can do these moves daily, but if that's not possible, aim to do them most days a week for the best results.

TIPPING BIRD

IMPROVES RANGE OF MOTION IN: Hamstrings, hips, and glutes

Stand tall with your arms out to the sides at shoulder height. Lift your right foot behind you, keeping your right leg extended, and balance on your left leg. Slowly hinge forward from the hips, tipping your torso forward toward the floor while extending your right leg straight behind you, foot flexed, until your body forms a straight line from your head to your heel. Stop when you're parallel to the floor. Return to the starting position. Switch sides. Alternate for a set of 10 on each side.

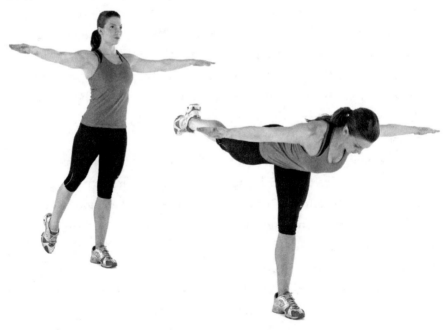

EXTENDED TRIANGLE

IMPROVES RANGE OF MOTION IN: Adductors
(inner thighs), abductors (outer thighs),
hips, obliques, glutes, and back

Step your feet 3½ to 4 feet apart, so you're in a wide straddle stance. Raise your arms and reach them out to the sides parallel to the floor with palms down. Turn your right foot in slightly to the left and your left foot out 90 degrees to the left. Keeping your arms extended, bend from the hip and extend your torso to the left directly over your left leg. Rest your left hand on the floor outside your left foot (or on your shin if you can't reach that far), while reaching toward the ceiling with your right hand. Turn your head to gaze up toward the right hand. Hold 30 seconds, then switch sides.

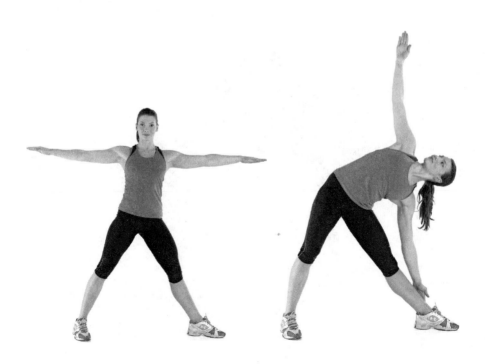

PYRAMID POSE

IMPROVES RANGE OF MOTION IN: Hamstrings, glutes, back, and shoulders

Step your feet $3^1/_2$ to 4 feet apart, so you're in a wide straddle stance. Pivot your body toward the right, so your feet are pointing in that direction and your hips are square. Turn your back foot out about 45 degrees. Keeping your hips squared and facing forward, lean forward at the hips and reach your hands down toward the floor, trying to place them on either side of your front foot. If you can't reach the floor, place your hands anywhere on your left leg for stability. (You can also place one hand on a chair or wall if balance is a challenge.) Hold 30 seconds. Then switch sides.

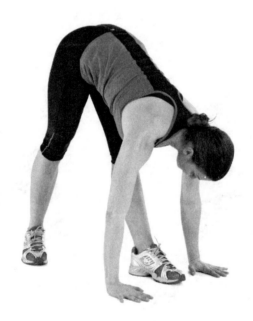

COBRA

Lie facedown with your feet together, toes pointed, and your hands on the floor, palms down just in front of your shoulders. Lift your chin and gently extend your arms, lifting your upper body off the floor as far as comfortably possible, while keeping your hips firmly anchored to the floor. If you feel any strain in your back, alter the pose so that you keep your elbows bent and forearms on the floor. Hold this position for 30 to 60 seconds.

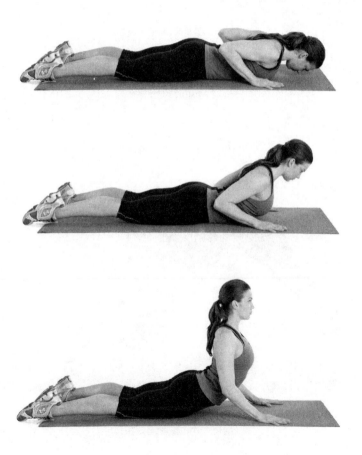

DOWNWARD DOG

IMPROVES RANGE OF MOTION IN: Hamstrings, calves, back, hips, and shoulders

Begin on your hands and knees. Place your feet hip width apart with toes tucked under. Place your hands shoulder width apart. Press into your palms and straighten your legs, lifting your tailbone toward the ceiling while pulling your navel toward your spine. Gently press your torso through your arms and your heels toward the floor. Hold this position for 30 to 60 seconds.

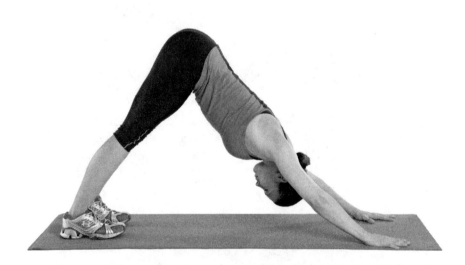

STABILITY BALL HIP FLEXOR STRETCH

IMPROVES RANGE OF MOTION IN: Hips, adductors, and quadriceps

Hold on to a chair back or tabletop for balance. Stand to the right and slightly to the front of an inflated stability ball and bend your left leg, placing your left shin and top of your left foot on the ball, so your leg is slightly extended (from the hip) behind you. Bend your right knee and extend your left leg back, pushing the ball away from you as you sink down into your hips. Hold 10 seconds. Switch legs. Perform 2 or 3 times per leg.

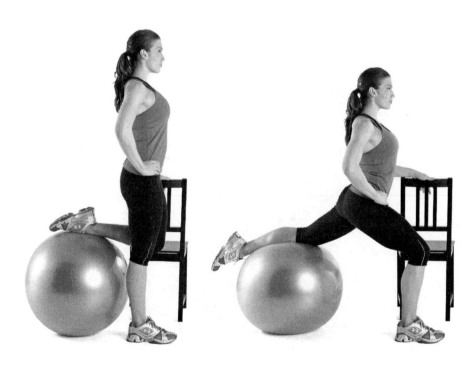

THIGH LENGTHENER

IMPROVES RANGE OF MOTION IN: Hips, quadriceps, and shins

Kneel on a carpeted floor or mat with your knees hip distance apart. Extend your arms in front of you, so they are straight out at shoulder height. Tuck your chin to your chest and lean your body back as far as comfortably possible while maintaining a straight line from your shoulders to your knees. Hold 5 to 10 seconds. Contract abdominal and glute muscles to bring your body back to the starting position. Perform 2 or 3 times.

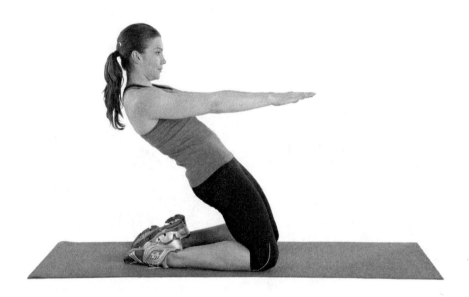

PIGEON

IMPROVES RANGE OF MOTION IN: Hips, quadriceps, glutes, shoulders, and chest

Start in a kneeling position, sitting on your heels. Keeping your left knee bent, stretch your right leg back to a half-split position. Place your right knee on the floor with your leg fully extended. Rest your left leg on the floor so your left foot is positioned in front of your right hip and your left thigh is resting on the floor (if possible), knee pointing at an angle to the left. Lift your head to look up at the ceiling. Place your palms down on the floor next to the left knee. Hold 30 seconds, then release. Switch legs.

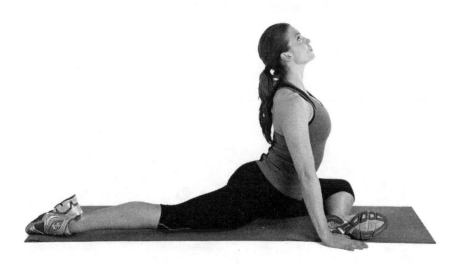

STRADDLE-SEATED WINDMILL

**IMPROVES RANGE OF MOTION IN: Hamstrings,
adductors, back, obliques, and hips**

Sit up tall on the floor with your back straight and legs extended and open wider than shoulder width apart. Extend your arms out to the sides at shoulder height. Twist to the right, reaching your left hand down to the outside of your right foot, while extending the right arm behind you. Hold 10 seconds, return to the center, and switch sides. Perform 2 or 3 times per leg.

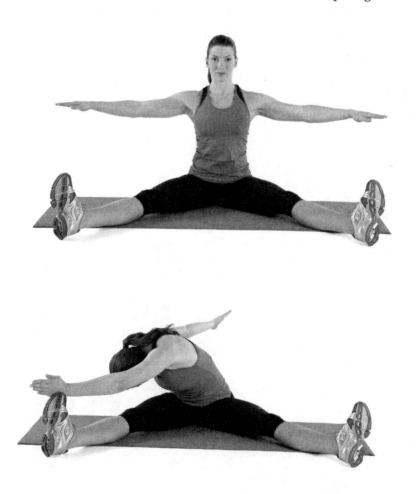

BACK BEND/CHEST OPENER

IMPROVES RANGE OF MOTION IN: Chest
and shoulders

Stand with your legs in a straddle stance. Place your hands behind your
back on your hips and press your fingertips together. Slowly work your
hands up your back as far as comfort allows, pressing your palms together,
if possible. Pivot your left foot and turn your body 90 degrees to the left.
The back foot should rotate a little less, remaining at a 45-degree angle to
provide better balance. Drop your shoulders and extend your chest, torso,
and hips. Tilt your head slightly back to look up toward the ceiling. Hold
10 seconds. Return to the starting position and switch sides. Perform 2
times per side.

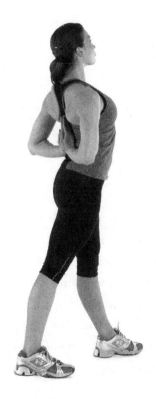

MIX IT UP

Even the most top-level pros dip their toes in other sports now and again. It helps them stay both mentally and physically well-rounded so they avoid burnout and imbalance. Cross-training not only gives you a break from the bike now and then but also provides options for burning fat and calories and keeps your weight-loss results rolling when you can't ride because of weather or travel.

There are countless ways to cross-train, from African dance classes at the Y to snowboarding in Brighton. Find something that speaks to you. Here are a few suggestions.

Swimming. Water is very forgiving of extra weight, so it's gentle on your joints and provides an excellent opportunity to stretch out and strengthen your core, upper back, and shoulder muscles while getting an amazing cardiovascular workout. It's one of the best exercises everyone can do.

Hiking. Nothing more than walking on a trail, hiking offers a challenge to your muscles and cardiovascular system (and scorches calories) while invigorating your senses and rejuvenating your mind. You don't need to live in Yosemite or close to the Appalachian Trail to do it, either. Any path through a park will do.

Walk/jogging. Running is pretty hard on the joints if you're carrying a lot of extra weight, especially if you're not accustomed to it. But, let's face it, it's a pretty convenient way to stay fit, because it burns several thousand calories an hour. Instead of pounding your knees into the ground trying to run continuously, try walk/jogging. Start with a brisk walk. Warm up for about 10 minutes. Then jog for 30 seconds. Return to a brisk walk for a few minutes, and then jog again. As you become more fit, increase the jogging time until you hit a few minutes.

Skiing. For riders who live in wintry climes, skiing, especially cross-country skiing, tops the list of cross-training sports that completely fry fat and keep your cycling muscles really strong. It also stretches your hip flexors and builds incredible cardiovascular endurance. Snowshoeing is another excellent option for those not coordinated on skis.

Strength-training. It counts as cross-training and is something you can and should do year-round to stay strong and balanced and keep your metabolism running high. Oh, and you're in luck, you have a plan right here! So no excuses. Get started today.

8:KEEPING IT OFF

ONCE THE WEIGHT IS GONE, KEEP IT GONE FOR GOOD

ANYONE WHO'S EVER managed to shrink down to a happier size will tell you that weight maintenance can be far harder than weight loss. Research shows that among people who lose a significant amount of weight, at least a third of them (some research says the percentage is even higher) will gain it all back and maybe more. That's true no matter how you lose it, including, in all honesty, if you ride it off. Some of it is behavioral. It's easy to grow a little complacent, ride a little less, dig a little less deep, and eat a little more. But basic biology is to blame as well. When you lose weight, your body tends to fight back with hunger and hormones to regain those pounds, which was a protective mechanism in times of famine, but is pretty counterproductive for most of us in modern times.

The good news is that scientists have been hard at work studying weight maintenance for decades, so now we have a pretty clear picture of what it takes to keep lost pounds off for good. It won't always be easy. But it will be worth it. By using your bike, it can also be a pretty enjoyable ride. Here's what you need to know.

✳RIDE LOTS

The National Weight Control Registry reports that successful "losers" exercise every day, doing 60 to 75 minutes of moderate exercise, like brisk walking, or 35 to 45 minutes of more vigorous exercise, like cycling. We know you can handle that. You already have.

This level of exercise is essential not only for the calorie burn (which is of primary importance) but also for the impact it has on your well-being, stress levels, appetite, and hormones. As mentioned earlier, when you lose weight, your body triggers a cascade of events to encourage you to put it back on. Though research is still needed, exercise seems to help blunt some of these defenses, especially the ones affecting appetite. Long-term regular exercise seems to help regulate leptin, a hormone responsible for turning off appetite. When people become overweight, they actually make more leptin, but they seem to lose leptin sensitivity, so they don't get the signals to stop eating. But over time, healthy diet, good exercise habits, and weight loss seem to help reset your leptin levels and thermostat, so you can maintain healthy levels at your new weight.

Regular riding also lowers your stress levels. That's important because when stress skyrockets, so does the hormone cortisol, which has a way of sending you straight for the cookie jar and transporting all those extra calories straight to your belly to be stored as dangerous, visceral fat. Riding your bike also improves your sense of self-efficacy, your sense of power to control a situation. It takes fitness and skill and effort to ride, especially to ride hard. Each time you do it, you increase your belief in yourself to make—and maintain—a positive change in your lifestyle. That goes a long way in keeping off weight.

CREATE AN ENERGY GAP

Whether you want to avoid gaining weight in the first place or prevent weight regain, you need to create an "energy gap," say obesity experts who have been studying how energy intake (calories in) relates to energy burn (calories out) and how it affects body weight. In plain terms, they have found that if you've lost a lot of weight (i.e., 10 percent or more of your body weight), you need to keep a constant energy gap—burn more than you take in—to keep it off. In the case of big losers, that energy gap needs to be 200 to 300 calories a day. This is especially important for riders in their forties and beyond, because as we age, our metabolism naturally dips, so we need fewer calories to maintain our weight, whether or not we've ever been overweight or lost weight.

Sounds like a lot. And it is. Three hundred calories is the amount in a small meal. But as long as you continue riding, as recommended above, it's actually quite manageable. In the Fit for Life plan, you'll continue riding and, most important, challenging yourself to go farther, faster, and try new things. This is important because your body adjusts to whatever activity level you give it. So if you're riding most days a week, that's your new activity level. To get the energy gap you need to keep the weight off, you need to do just that little bit extra. To guarantee your success, combine your riding with a little trimming of your portion sizes to eliminate about 150 calories, an amount that's far easier to swallow, if you'll pardon the pun, than 300. Here are a few easy ways to trim 150 calories from your daily diet.

Wrap it up. One sandwich wrap generally has the same amount of calories as a single slice of bread. A far better choice for your sandwich needs.

Skip the soft drinks. They add nothing but weight.

Leave bites behind. If you leave just a few bites behind at every meal, you can be a bit less vigilant about what's on your plate.

Spread less. Whether it's butter or mayo, use a tablespoon or knifeful less. Better yet, try using mustard instead; it's very low in fat and calories.

Choose Canadian. Canadian bacon has far fewer calories than the regular kind.

Have it on the rocks. Treat yourself to that cocktail on the rocks. Frozen drinks are filled with sugary syrups. Or order a white wine spritzer—the seltzer and ice will make it last longer.

Skip the cheese. Just one slice of cheese left behind will help keep those pounds behind too.

Go for grilled. Fried anything is going to have at least 150 more calories than the grilled version.

Banish "breaded." Breading adds calories you don't need, and it's usually fried, adding even more.

Rediscover coffee. What did we do before calorie-laden Frappuccinos? We drank coffee, and it didn't feel like much of a sacrifice because it's actually pretty good, even without the whipped cream.

✳ WEIGH IN

It's easier to lose 3 pounds than it is 10. Though no one should be a slave to the scale, the vast majority of people who keep the weight off step on the scale at least once a week.

It's not a fun ritual, but it's one that will help make you be accountable to yourself for your actions (riding and eating smartly), which in itself helps keep unwanted weight from making a comeback. The easiest approach is to weigh yourself at about the same time each week. Monday morning is a good time, because it's like New Year's Day of each week, a time when you may have indulged a little over the weekend and need to get back on track for the days ahead.

Record your weight in your workout log. Allow for small fluctuations of a pound or two. But once you see the numbers trending northward by 3 pounds or more, it's time to regroup, pay attention to portions, and make sure you're getting in quality rides complete with metabolism-revving intervals.

✳ TUNE OUT

Want an easy way to create about half that energy gap we talked about earlier? Push "off" on the TV remote. Most Americans watch an average of 5 hours of television a day, third only to time spent sleeping and working. It is also the single most sedentary activity you can do short of sleeping. Zoning out in front of the TV burns fewer calories than reading, working at your desk, writing, and talking on the phone.

Little surprise then that the number of hours you spend sitting in front of a screen, especially a television screen, has a strong correlation to the number of notches in your belt, and that numerous studies have linked TV watching to a high risk for weight gain. You're almost always sitting, and very often eating, whenever the tube is on.

Fortunately, the opposite is also true. When the tube is powered down, your body tends to be in motion, according to a recent intervention study published in the *Archives of Internal Medicine*. The researchers observed the activity and eating habits of 36 overweight men and women who watched an average of 5 hours of television a day for 3 weeks. Then, using special monitors, they limited the amount of time half the group could watch TV to 2½ hours—a 50 percent decrease—and monitored everyone for another 3 weeks. At the end of the study, they found that those who halved their TV-watching time still ate the same amount of food but burned 120 more calories a day—the equivalent of walking about 1¼ miles.

One easy way to slice your screen time: invest in TiVo or another digital recording device. That way you can watch only what you want to watch when you want to watch it and zip through the commercials, so you can enjoy your favorite shows in less time.

✳ GET CONNECTED

True, you can always ride alone. But let's face it: it's more fun with a friend. You're also far more likely to bundle up in the cold, bear a little wind or drizzle, and set the alarm extra early when you know a friend awaits.

There are myriad ways to get connected with like-minded cyclists. One of the best ways is joining a local cycling club (the Internet is a good source for organizations in your area). Cycling clubs aren't just for racers. They're filled with people just like you who want a little camaraderie out there on the roads and trails. They often hold weekly rides for cyclists of all experience and fitness levels as well as travel together to organized rides, charity events, and races. You also can swing into your local bike shop and ask about organized rides that leave from there. Most bike shops have "shop rides," where locals meet at a certain time each week and spin out for a designated amount of time.

You can also connect yourself to the cycling community, and dedicate all your hard work to the greater good, by participating in charity rides like the MS 150 (a popular 2-day, 150-mile ride that benefits multiple sclerosis treatment and research). Having a goal ride to shoot for will also help keep you motivated to maintain—or even improve—your cycling fitness. Plus, you're sure to meet more riders just like you.

Glenn Allen, 33, of Phoenix, Arizona, discovered you can find groups right in your backyard that you never knew existed . . . and they can take you places you never imagined. "I had been a recreational rider years ago, but then I went to graduate school and got a job and had two kids and basically stopped riding. My weight swelled up to 245 pounds, and I'm 5'9". In July of 2007, I decided that I'd had enough." Glenn went out and bought a Trek 5.2 Madone. But the ride back was much harder than he expected. "I was dying. I could barely ride 20 miles, which makes sense when you consider how heavy I was, but I had a hard time reconciling it with what I knew I used to be able to do."

Glenn persisted, and some friends convinced him to ride the 66-mile El Tour de Tucson later that year. "I had to stop twice," he recalls. But he whittled his weight down to 197. He sold the Trek, did a few months of running over the winter (lost more weight), and bought an Orbea Orca in spring of 2008. He searched the Internet to find more people to ride with and located a group right by his house that rode every weekend. He rode every weekend, outgrew that group, and found another, faster circle of riders, also close by. Before he knew it he was doing Tuesday night criterium races as well as hard weekend rides. His weight hit 155 pounds. He did El Tour de Tucson again this year and finished sixth—in a sprint for the finish. "Just 2 years ago, I couldn't sprint down the block," he says with a laugh. "Now I'm more of a cycling enthusiast than ever before!"

✳KEEP IT CONVENIENT

When you first start riding a lot and watching the pounds come off, you're bound to be brimming with enthusiasm and willing to make all sorts of sacrifices to get out on your bike as often as possible. Once you've reached your goal and the honeymoon begins to fade, however, excuses can start to creep in. Keeping riding as convenient as possible will help nip them in the bud before they keep you off your bike.

Take it from Ray Adams, 50, from South Bay Beach Cities, California, who bought a mountain bike to get back in shape. "I started out weighing 200 pounds and gradually started increasing the length and frequency of my rides. I used to rush home from work to get in an hour of saddle time before dinner," he recalls, noting that it wasn't long before all that dashing around was just too hectic to maintain. "So I switched to mornings before work. After a year of riding the mountain bike, I realized I wanted to go faster, so I bought my first real road bike. I now ride 5 to 6 days a week, 20 to 30 miles a day during the week; 40 to 60 on weekend days, averaging about 200 miles a week." He not only has held steady at a healthy 170 pounds but also enjoys a much more stable disposition. "I don't get as upset as I used to get. Things that used to get me fired up rarely get me worked up anymore. I recommend riding to lose weight, control your weight, and help with your mental health!"

Make it easy to get out and ride by picking a time of day when you have a little buffer zone and don't need to feel terribly rushed. Keep all your cycling gear in one easy-to-access place, so you can get dressed, fill your bottles, grab your shoes, helmet, gloves, and go. Little tricks like laying out your cycling clothes the night before go a long way in helping you stay on track day to day.

BE MORE NEAT

Regular riding is important, but simple daily activity known as NEAT (*non-exercise activity thermogenesis*) is equally essential for a healthy metabolism. Small daily movements like stretching your legs, taking the stairs, even just standing to talk on the phone can add up to an additional 350 calories burned a day—hello, energy gap (are you sensing a trend here?).

Here are some simple daily swaps you can make to get off your glutes and keep your metabolism humming along on high.

INSTEAD OF . . .	DO THIS . . .	BURN . . .
Sitting at your desk	Stand to work	35 more cals per hr
Calling for delivery	Whip up a quick meal at home	70 more cals per hr
Riding the elevator	Take the stairs	410 more cals per hr
Shopping online	Head downtown (or to the mall)	55 more cals per hr
Hiring a lawn service	Mow the lawn	270 more cals per hr
Watching TV sitting	Stretch or do yoga while you watch	100 more cals per hr
E-mailing a co-worker	Stroll to his/her office	35 more cals per hr
Renting a movie	Go to an art opening	55 more cals per hr
Opening the back door	Walk the dog	100 more cals per hr
Playing video games	Play tennis or go bowling/fishing	135 more cals per hr
Surfing the Web	Visit a museum	55 more cals per hr

SECRETS OF LONG-TERM LOSERS

- 90 percent exercise about an hour a day
- 78 percent eat breakfast every day
- 75 percent step on the scale once a week
- 62 percent watch fewer than 10 hours of TV per week

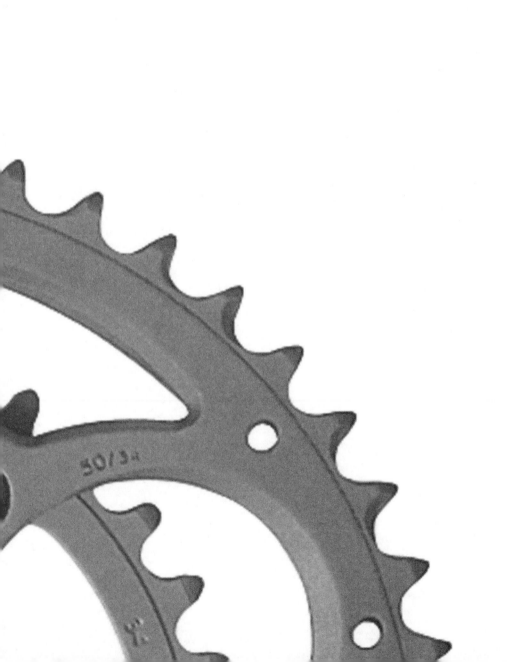

INDEX

Underscored page references indicate tables or shaded text.